An Atlas of
Radiological Interpretation
The Bones

An Atlas of

Radiological Interpretation

The Bones

John F Calder

MB ChB, FRCR
Consultant Radiologist
Victoria Infirmary, Glasgow

Gwen Chessell

Dip Ed Tech, M Ed
Coordinator, Medical Learning Resources Group
University of Aberdeen

Wolfe Medical Publications Limited

For a full list of other titles published by Wolfe Medical Publications Ltd,
please write to the publishers at Brook House, 2–16 Torrington Place,
London WC1E 7LT, England.

Contents

Acknowledgements

We wish to thank those colleagues, past and present, who have contributed to the X-ray film libraries of Aberdeen Royal Infirmary, the Kenyatta National Hospital, Nairobi and the Victoria Infirmary, Glasgow. We also wish to thank the staff of the Department of Medical Illustration, University of Aberdeen, who have helped to reproduce the radiographs.

We would like to mention especially:
Dr A P Bayliss
Dr J S H Davidson
Professor L A Gillanders
Dr J K Hussey
Dr A F MacDonald
Dr R G Mahaffy
Dr E M Robertson
Dr F W Smith
Dr E J Stockdale
Dr P R Ward
Dr J Weir
Professor L R Whittaker
Mrs R Horberry

Introduction

The idea for this atlas evolved from a series of teaching slides produced for individual study programmes developed for the Learning Resources Area of Aberdeen University Medical School Library. The radiographs used have formed the basis of courses given to undergraduates and to postgraduates reading for the qualifications of D.M.R.D. (Aberdeen) and M.Med. Radiology (Nairobi).

The atlas includes most of the common conditions seen in everyday radiological practice, as well as some rarer examples which should be of particular interest to students and doctors.

1: NORMAL ANATOMY

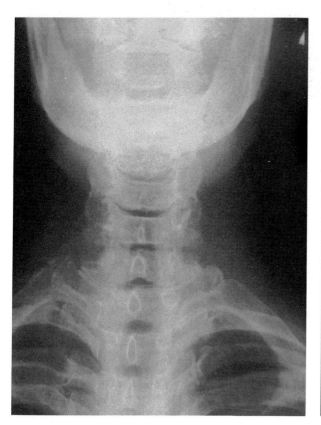
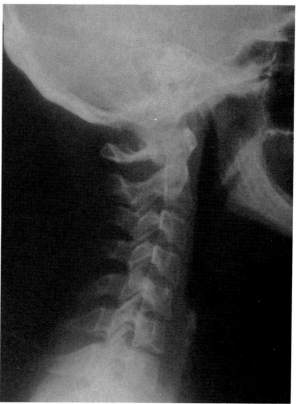

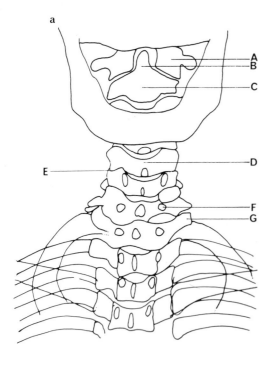
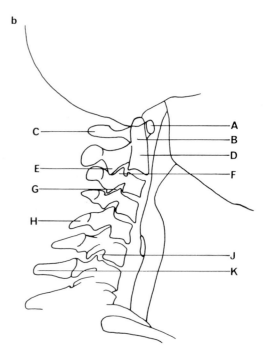

a

A
B
C
D
E
F
G

b

C
A
B
D
E
F
G
H
J
K

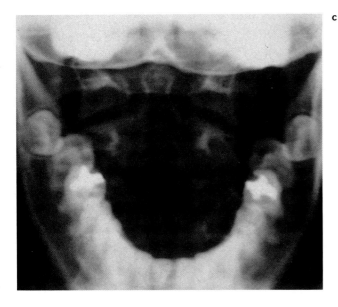
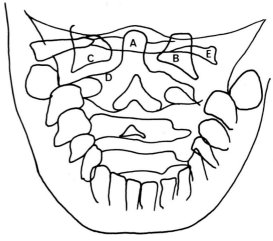

1(c) AP atlas and axis.
  A   Odontoid process of C2
  B   Lateral mass of C1
  C   Inferior articular surface of C1
  D   Superior articular surface of C2
  E   Transverse process of C1

1(a) AP cervical spine.
◀ A   Lateral mass of Cl (atlas)
  B   Odontoid process of C2 (axis)
  C   Body of C2
  D   Body of C4
  E   C4/5 apophyseal joint
  F   Pedicle of C7
  G   Transverse process of T1

1(b) Lateral cervical spine.
◀ A   Anterior arch of C1
  B   Odontoid process of C2
  C   Posterior arch of C1
  D   Body of C2
  E   Inferior articular process of C2
  F   Superior articular process of C3
  G   C3/4 apophyseal joint
  H   Spinous process of C5
  J   C6/7 intervertebral foramen
  K   Spinous process of C7 (vertebra prominens)

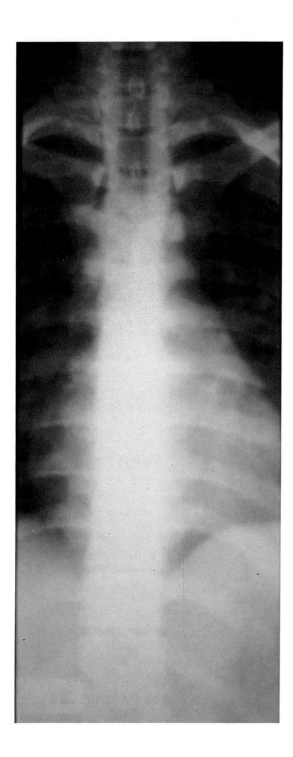

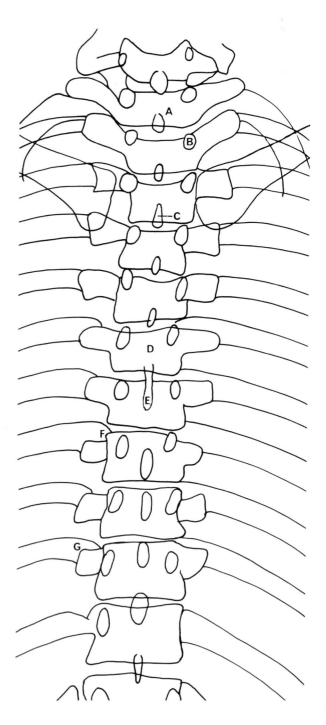

2(a) **AP thoracic spine.**
A Body of T1
B Pedicle of T2
C Spinous process of T3
D Body of T6
E Spinous process of T6
F Costo-vertebral joint of T8
G Costo-transverse joint of T9

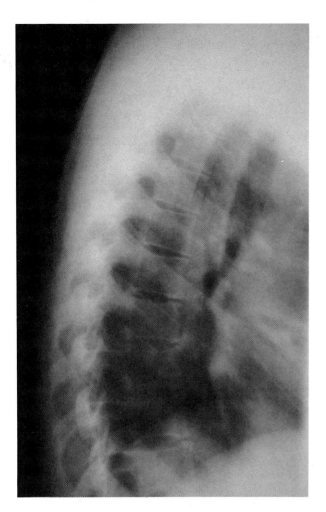

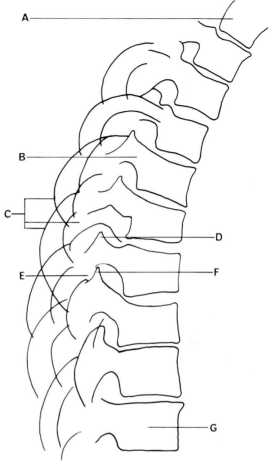

2(b) Lateral thoracic spine.
  A   Body of T2
  B   Lamina of T6
  C   Ribs
  D   Superior articular process of T8
  E   Inferior articular process of T8
  F   T8/9 apophyseal joint
  G   Body of T11

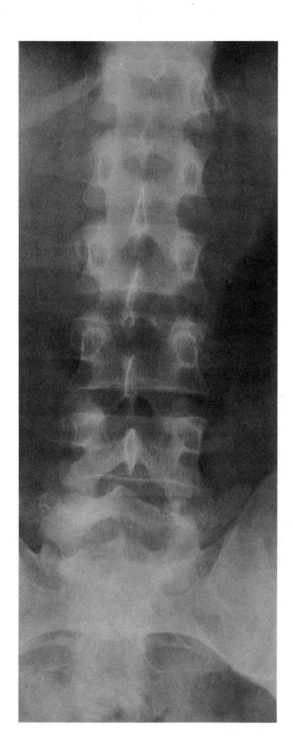
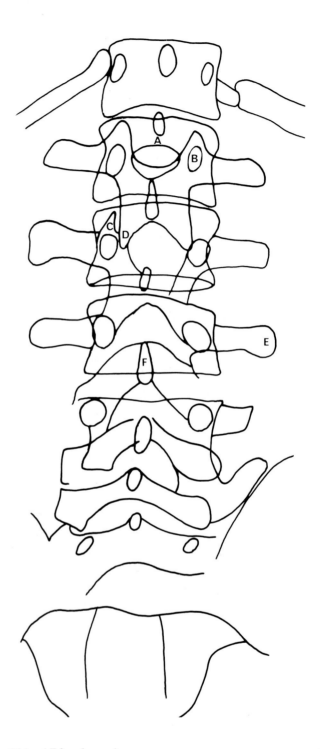

3(a) AP lumbar spine.
A   Body of L1
B   Pedicle of L1
C   Superior articular process of L2
D   Inferior articular process of L1
E   Transverse process of L3
F   Spinous process of L3

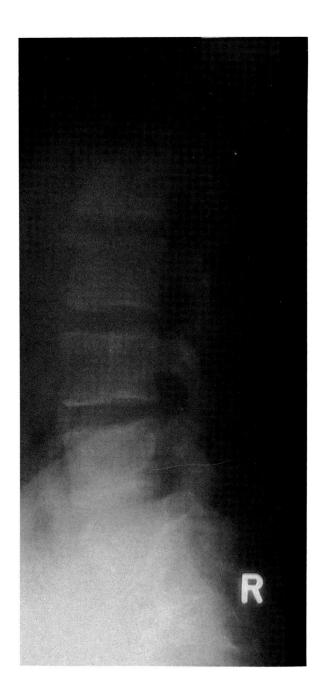

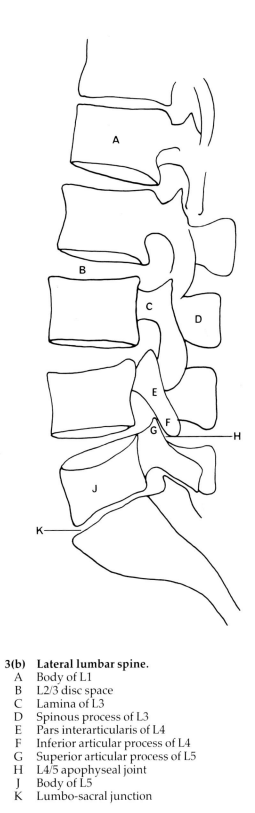

3(b) Lateral lumbar spine.
A   Body of L1
B   L2/3 disc space
C   Lamina of L3
D   Spinous process of L3
E   Pars interarticularis of L4
F   Inferior articular process of L4
G   Superior articular process of L5
H   L4/5 apophyseal joint
J   Body of L5
K   Lumbo-sacral junction

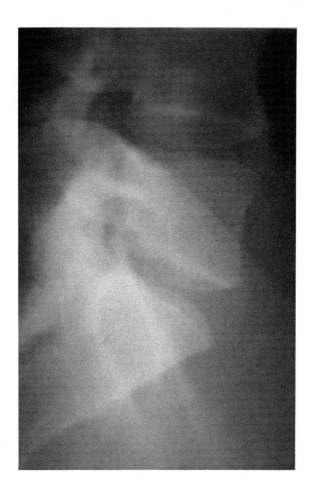

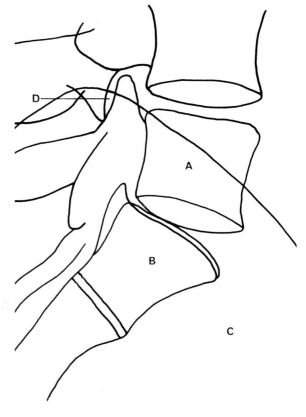

3(c) **Lateral lumbo-sacral angle.**
  A   Body of L5
  B   Body of S1
  C   Ilium
  D   L4/5 apophyseal joint

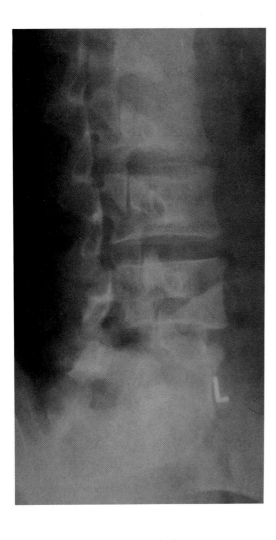

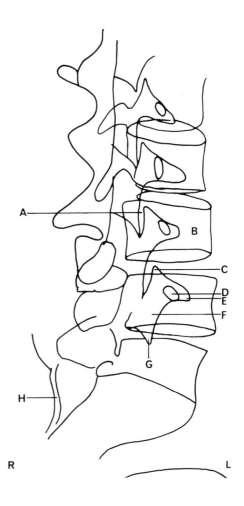

3(d) Right anterior oblique lumbar spine.
A   Left L3/4 apophyseal joint
B   Body of L4
C   Left superior articular process of L5
D   Left pedicle of L5
E   Left transverse process of L5
F   Left pars interarticularis of L5
G   Left inferior articular process of L5
The appearances of C to G have been likened to a 'Scottie dog'. The ear is the superior articular process, the eye is the pedicle, the nose is the transverse process, the neck is the pars interarticularis and the foreleg is the inferior articular facet.
H   Right sacro-iliac joint

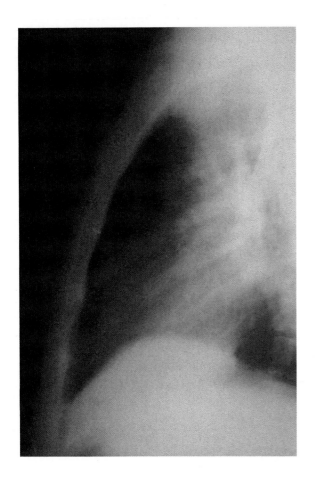

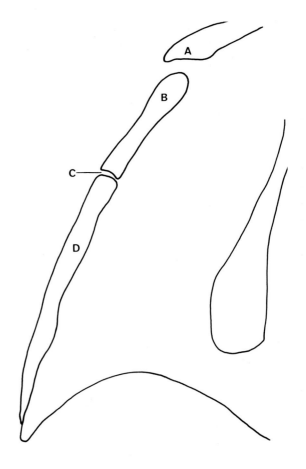

4 **Lateral sternum.**
  A   Clavicle
  B   Manubrium
  C   Manubrio-sternal joint (sternal angle)
  D   Sternum

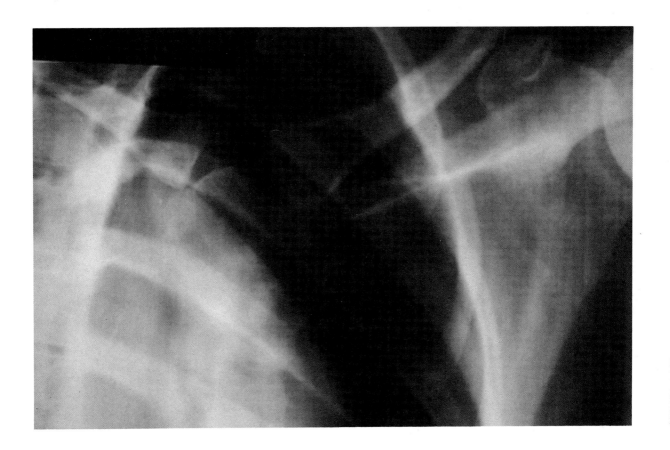

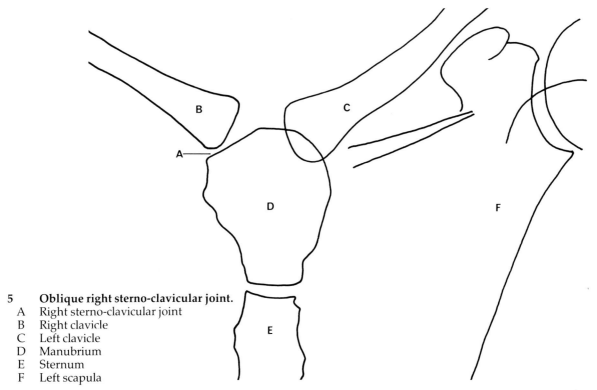

5   **Oblique right sterno-clavicular joint.**
  A   Right sterno-clavicular joint
  B   Right clavicle
  C   Left clavicle
  D   Manubrium
  E   Sternum
  F   Left scapula

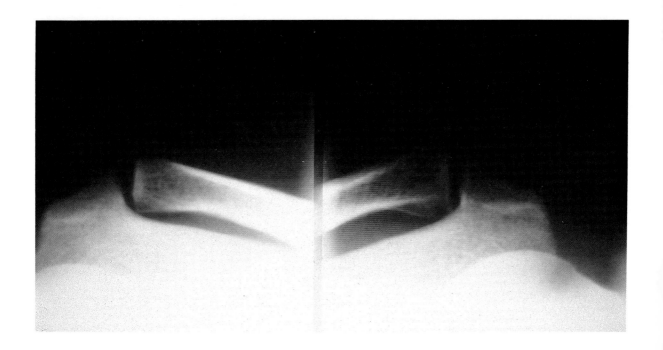

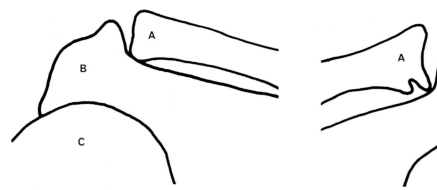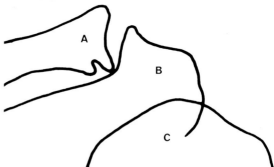

6   Acromio-clavicular joints.
  A   Clavicle
  B   Acromion
  C   Head of humerus

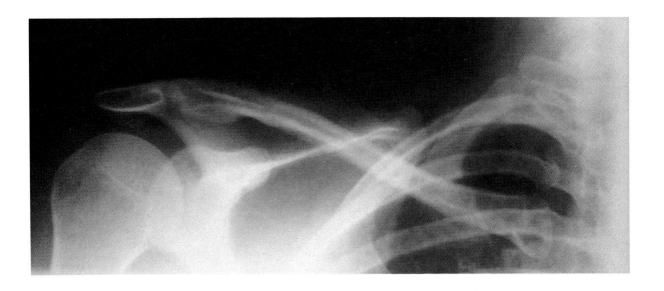

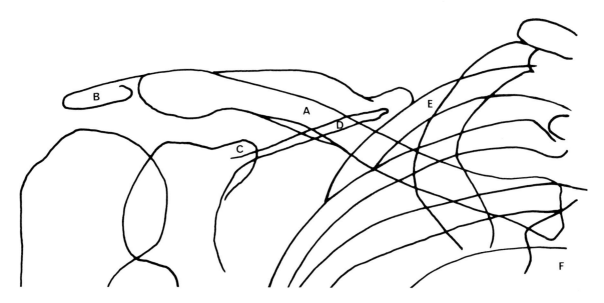

7   **Right clavicle.**
  A   Clavicle
  B   Acromion process of scapula
  C   Coracoid process of scapula
  D   Spine of scapula
  E   Ribs
  F   Manubrium

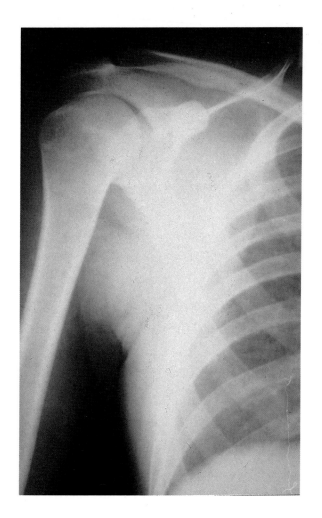

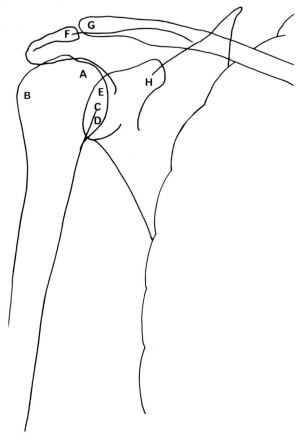

8(a) AP right shoulder.
A   Head of humerus
B   Greater tuberosity
C   Intertubercular sulcus
D   Lesser tuberosity of humerus
E   Glenoid process of scapula
F   Acromion process of scapula
G   Clavicle
H   Coracoid process of scapula

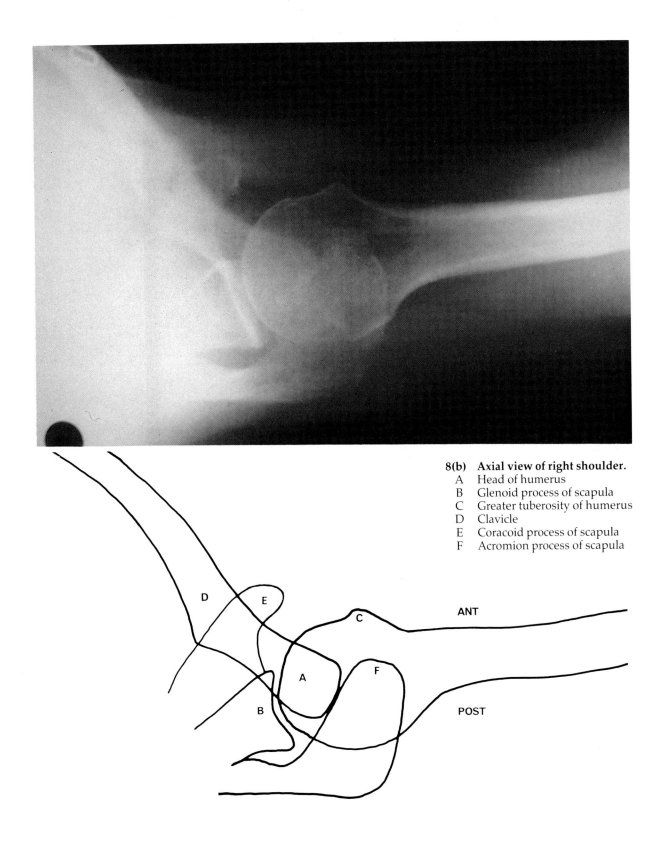

8(b) Axial view of right shoulder.
A Head of humerus
B Glenoid process of scapula
C Greater tuberosity of humerus
D Clavicle
E Coracoid process of scapula
F Acromion process of scapula

ANT

POST

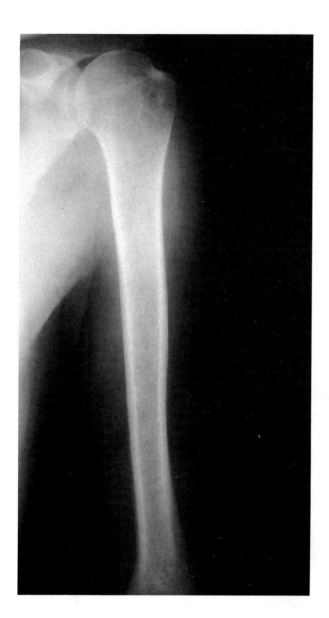
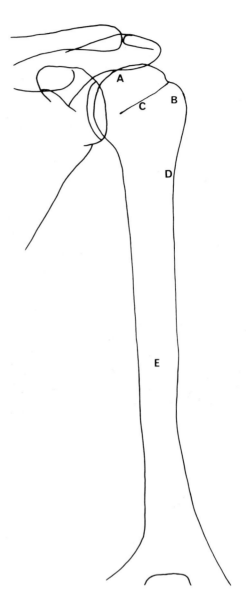

9   AP left humerus.
A   Head
B   Greater tuberosity
C   Anatomical neck
D   Surgical neck
E   Shaft

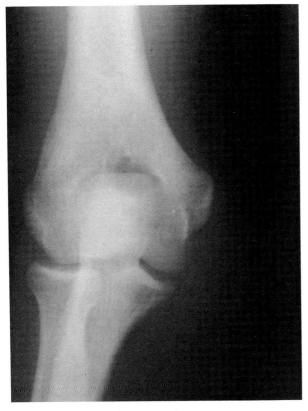

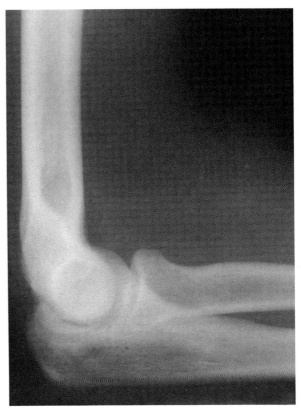

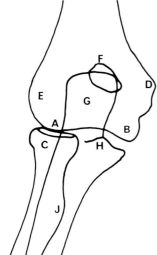

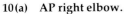

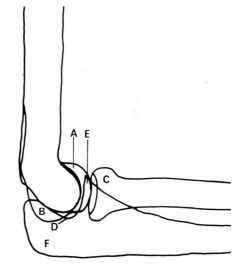

10(a) **AP right elbow.**
 A   Capitulum of humerus
 B   Trochlea of humerus
 C   Head of radius
 D   Medial epicondyle of humerus
 E   Lateral epicondyle of humerus
 F   Olecranon fossa of humerus
 G   Olecranon process of ulna
 H   Coronoid process of ulna
 J   Radial tuberosity

10(b) **Lateral right elbow.**
 A   Capitulum of humerus
 B   Trochlea of humerus
 C   Head of radius
 D   Sigmoid fossa of ulna
 E   Coronoid process of ulna
 F   Olecranon process of ulna

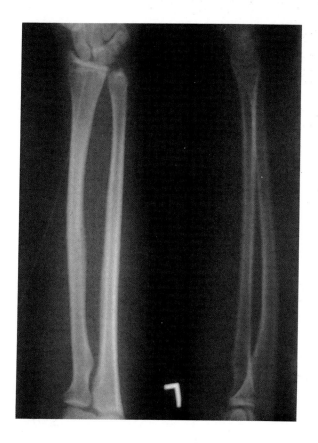
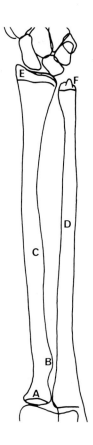
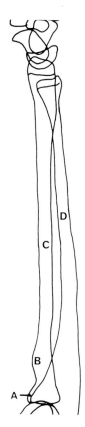

11   AP and lateral left forearm.
  A   Head of radius
  B   Radial tuberosity
  C   Radial shaft
  D   Ulnar shaft
  E   Radial styloid
  F   Ulnar styloid

12(a)   PA wrist and carpus.▶
  A   Radial styloid
  B   Ulnar styloid
  C   Scaphoid
  D   Lunate
  E   Triquetral
  F   Pisiform
  G   Trapezium
  H   Trapezoid
  J   Capitate
  K   Hamate
  L   Hook of hamate
  M   First metacarpal

12(b)   Lateral wrist and carpus.▶
  A   Radial styloid
  B   Ulnar styloid
  C   Scaphoid
  D   Lunate
  E   Triquetral
  G   Trapezium
  J   Capitate
  K   Hamate
  M   First metacarpal

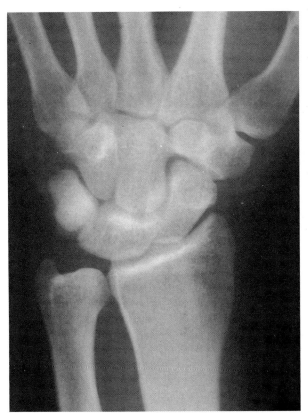

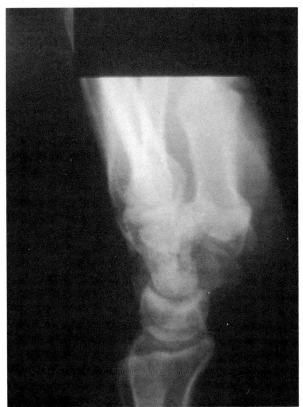

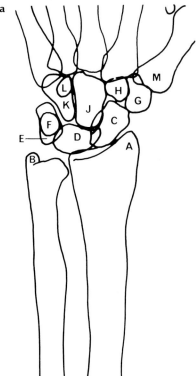

a

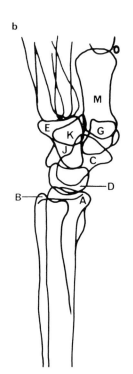

b

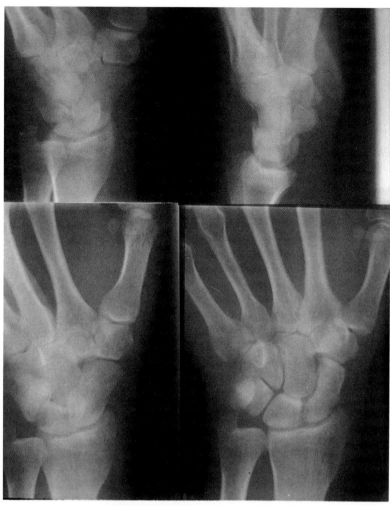

13   Scaphoid views.

(a) *PA*
(b) *Lateral*
(c) *Oblique*
(d) *Oblique*

A   Radial styloid
B   Ulnar styloid
C   Scaphoid
W   Waist of scaphoid
D   Lunate
E   Triquetral
F   Pisiform
G   Trapezium
H   Trapezoid
J   Capitate
K   Hamate
L   Hook of hamate
M   First metacarpal

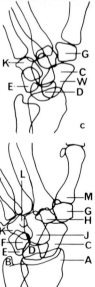

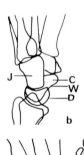

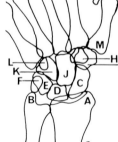

26

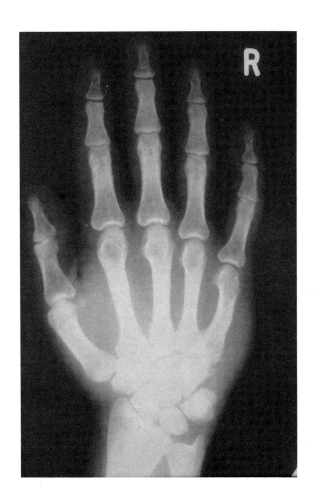

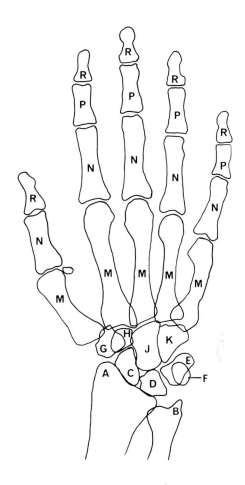

14   PA right hand.
A   Radial styloid
B   Ulnar styloid
C   Scaphoid
D   Lunate
E   Triquetral
F   Pisiform
G   Trapezium
H   Trapezoid
J   Capitate
K   Hamate
M   Metacarpals
N   Proximal phalanges
P   Middle phalanges
R   Distal phalanges

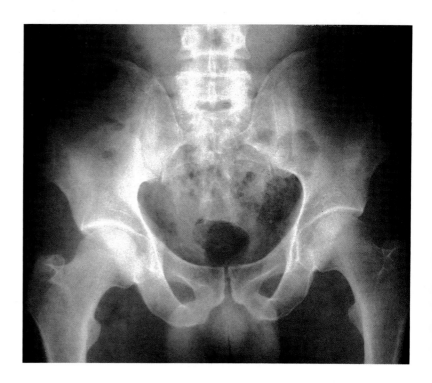

15   AP pelvis.

(a) Male

- A   Iliac crest
- B   Anterior superior iliac spine
- C   Anterior inferior iliac spine
- D   Pelvic brim
- E   Sacro-iliac joint
- F   Sacro-sciatic notch
- G   Ischial spine
- H   Superior pubic ramus
- J   Obdurator foramen
- K   Inferior ischial ramus
- L   Inferior pubic ramus
- M   Body of pubis
- N   Pubic symphysis
- P   Sub-pubic arch
- R   Acetabulum
- S   Head of femur
- T   Neck of femur
- V   Greater trochanter of femur
- W   Lesser trochanter of femur

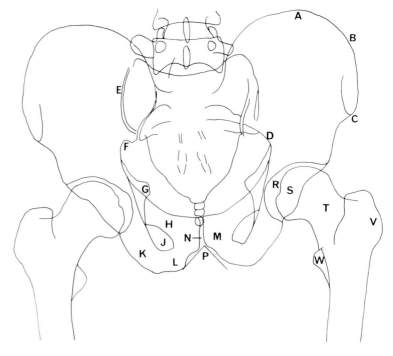

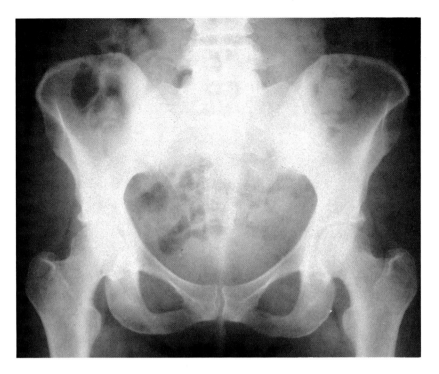

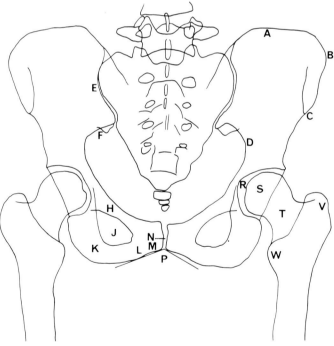

(b) Female
The annotation is the same as for the male pelvis.

Note: G (ischial spine), is not seen as it is much less prominent in the female.

Other differences in the female pelvis are:
D   a more rounded
    pelvic brim
F   a wider and
    shallower sacro-iliac
    notch
P   a wider sub-pubic
    arch and a curved
    sacrum, concave
    anteriorly (not
    shown).

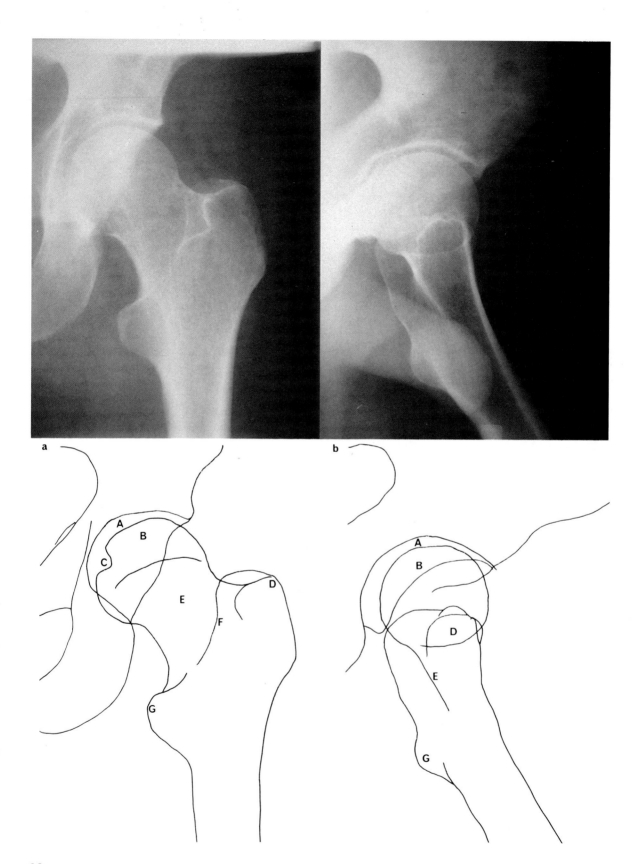

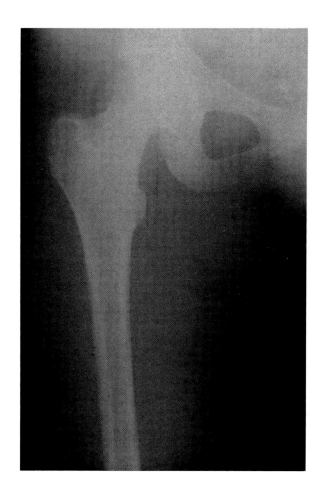

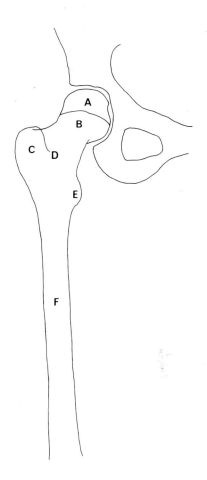

16(a) AP left hip.
◄ A Acetabulum
   B Femoral head
   C Fovea centralis
   D Greater trochanter
   E Femoral neck
   F Intertrochanteric line
   G Lesser trochanter

16(b) Lateral left hip.
◄ A Acetabulum
   B Femoral head
   D Greater trochanter
   E Femoral neck
   G Lesser trochanter

17   AP right femur.
   A Femoral head
   B Femoral neck
   C Greater trochanter
   D Intertrochanteric line
   E Lesser trochanter
   F Femoral shaft

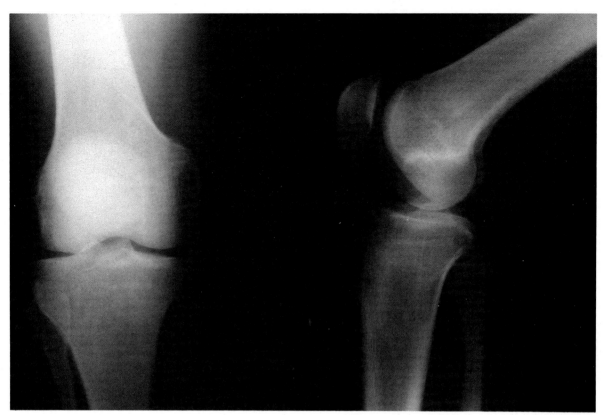

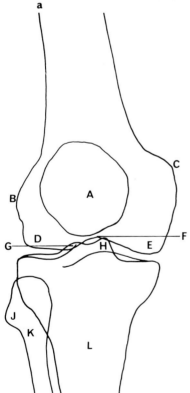

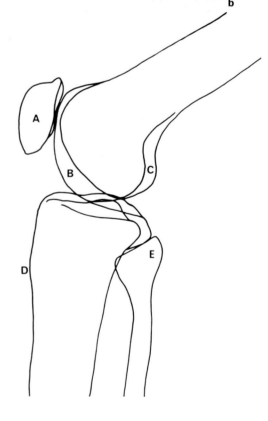

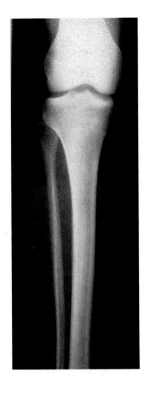
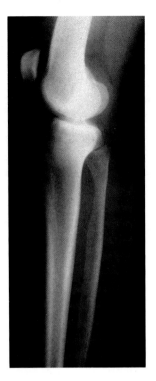
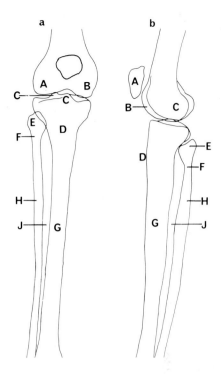

18(a) AP right knee.

◀ A Patella
  B Lateral epicondyle of femur
  C Medial epicondyle of femur
  D Lateral condyle of femur
  E Medial condyle of femur
  F Intercondylar notch
  G Lateral tibial spine
  H Medial tibial spine
  J Head of fibula
  K Neck of fibula
  L Tibia

18(b) Lateral right knee.

◀ A Patella
  B Medial femoral condyle
  C Lateral femoral condyle
  D Tibial tuberosity
  E Fibular head

19(a) AP right tibia and fibula.

  A Lateral femoral condyle
  B Medial femoral condyle
  C Tibial spines
  D Tibial tuberosity
  E Head of fibula
  F Neck of fibula
  G Shaft of tibia
  H Shaft of fibula
  J Interosseous membrane

19(b) Lateral right tibia and fibula.

  A Patella
  B Medial femoral condyle
  C Lateral femoral condyle
  D Tibial tuberosity
  E Head of fibula
  F Neck of fibula
  G Shaft of tibia
  H Shaft of fibula
  J Interosseous membrane

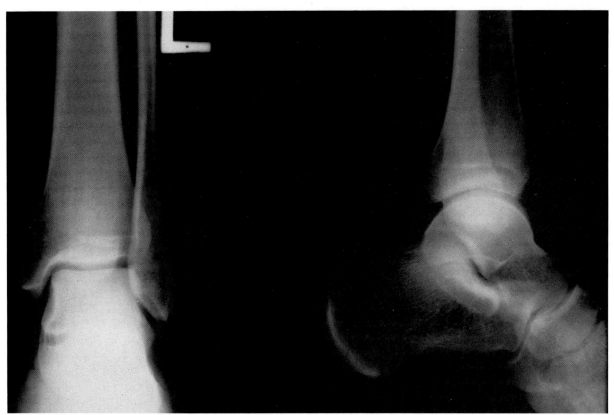

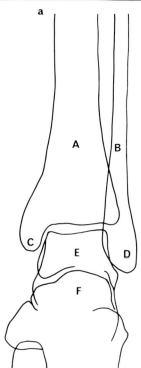

a

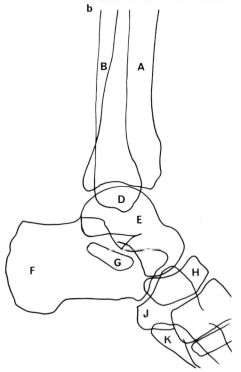

b

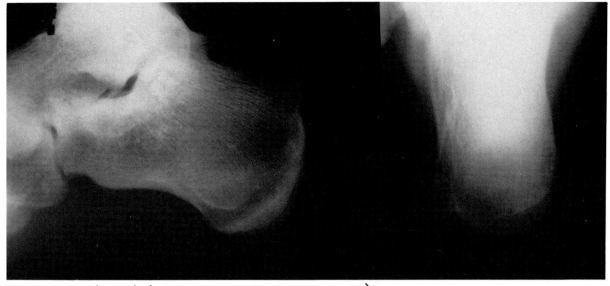

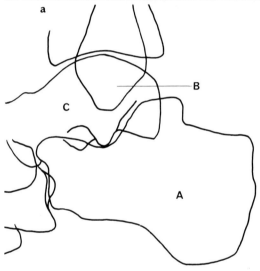

a

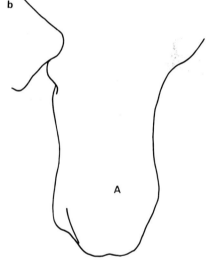

b

20(a)   AP left ankle.
◄ A   Tibia
  B   Fibula
  C   Medial malleolus
  D   Lateral malleolus
  E   Talus
  F   Calcaneus

20(b)   Lateral left ankle.
◄ A   Tibia
  B   Fibula
  D   Lateral malleolus
  E   Talus
  F   Calcaneus
  G   Sustentaculum tali
  H   Navicular
  J   Cuboid
  K   5th metatarsal

21(a)   Lateral left calcaneus.
  A   Calcaneus
  B   Lateral malleolus
  C   Talus

21(b)   Axial left calcaneus.
  A   Calcaneus

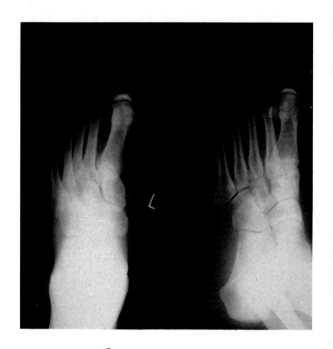

22(a) PA left foot.
22(b) Oblique left foot.
    A   Calcaneus
    B   Talus
    C   Cuboid
    D   Navicular
    E   Medial cuneiform
    F   Intermediate cuneiform
    G   Lateral cuneiform
    H   Metatarsals
    J   Proximal phalanges
    K   Middle phalanges
    L   Distal phalanges

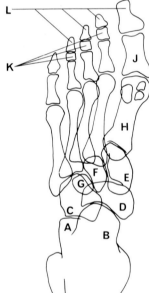

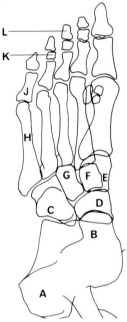

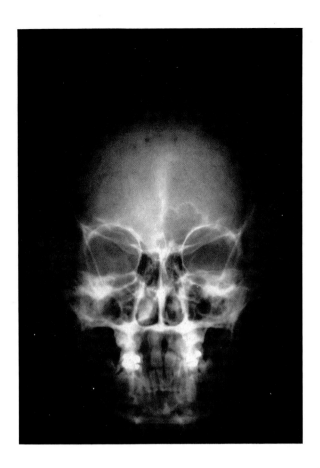

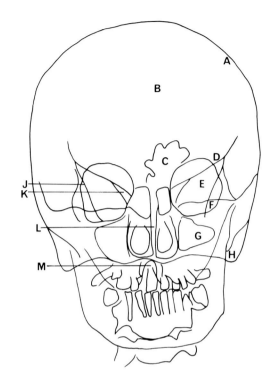

23 (a) PA skull.
    A   Parietal bone
    B   Frontal bone
    C   Frontal sinus
    D   Sphenoid ridge
    E   Greater wing of sphenoid
    F   Petrous ridge
    G   Maxillary antrum
    H   Mastoid process
    J   Innominate line
    K   Superior orbital fissure
    L   Nasal septum
    M   Odontoid

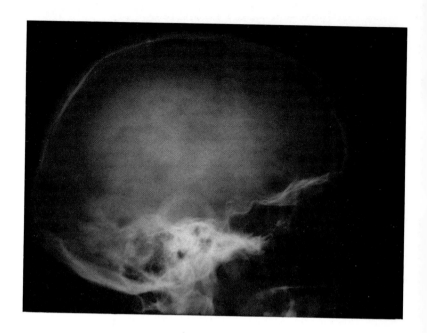

23(b)   Lateral skull.
  A   Frontal bone
  B   Coronal suture
  C   Parietal bone
  D   Lambdoid suture
  E   Occipital bone
  F   Mastoid air cells
  G   Pinna of ear
  H   External auditory meatus
  J   Temporo-mandibular
      joint
  K   Sphenoid sinus
  L   Maxillary antra
  M   Orbit
  N   Frontal sinuses
  P   Sella turcica

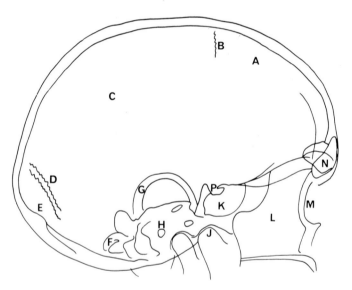

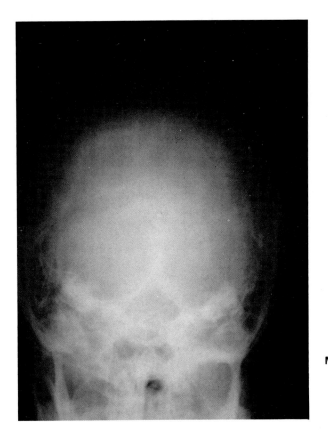

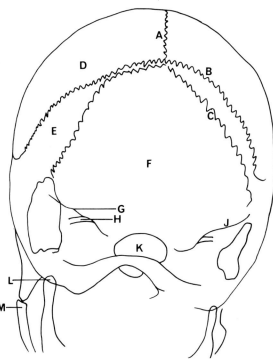

23 (c)   Towne's view of skull.
  A   Sagittal suture
  B   Coronal suture
  C   Lambdoid suture
  D   Parietal bone
  E   Frontal bone
  F   Occipital bone
  G   Arcuate eminence
  H   Internal auditory meatus
  J   Petrous ridge
  K   Foramen magnum
  L   Mandibular condyle
  M   Zygomatic arch

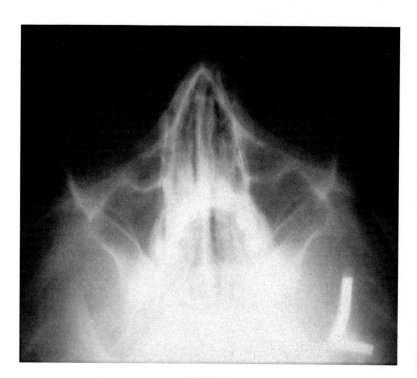

24 **Paranasal sinuses—occipito-mental view.**
A   Frontal sinus
B   Ethmoid sinuses
C   Maxillary sinus
D   Sphenoid sinus
E   Zygomatic arch
F   Orbit
G   Nasal septum

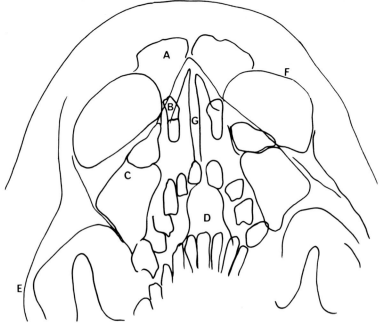

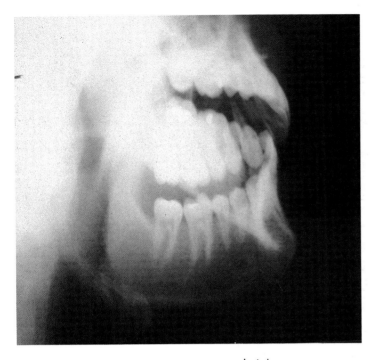

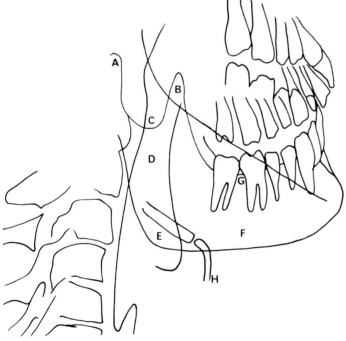

25 **Mandible—oblique view.**
A Mandibular condyle
B Coronoid process
C Mandibular notch
D Ramus
E Angle
F Body
G Alveolar border
H Hyoid bone

2: BONE TRAUMA

Trauma to bone is one of the most common problems in clinical and radiological practice. Fractures range in severity from trivial to life-threatening. As well as being important in themselves, fractures in certain sites such as the skull, the thoracic cage and pelvis may be associated with damage to adjacent viscera.

Many common fractures and dislocations, as well as some rarer ones, are shown in the following examples.

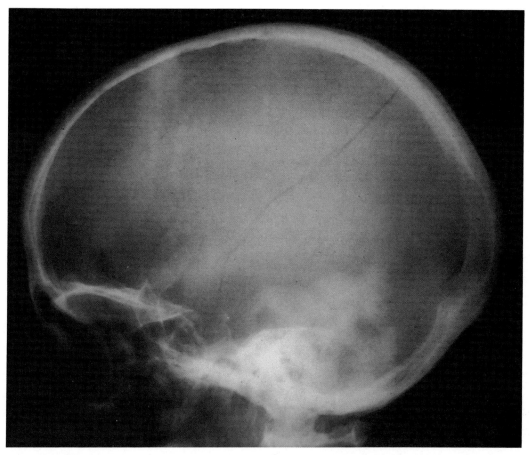

26 Skull fracture.
There is a linear fracture (A) of the parietal and temporal bones. Such fractures are not always associated with significant brain injury but do raise the possibility that one is present. In this case, there was an associated temporal lobe laceration.

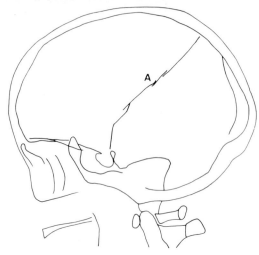

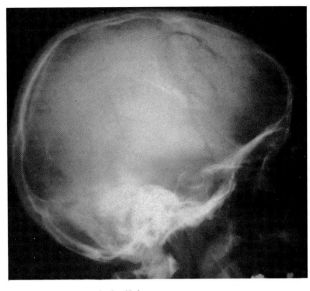
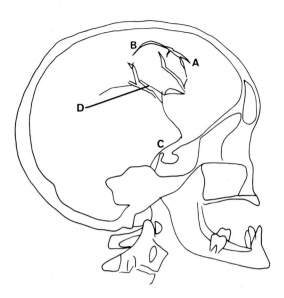

27   Depressed skull fracture.

(a) *Lateral view.*
Several left frontal (A), parietal (B) and
temporal (C) fracture lines can be seen.
There are double densities (D) in the
parietal bone indicating bony overlap
and hence depression.

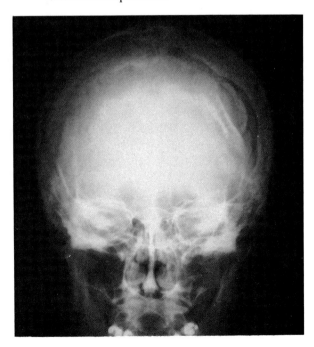
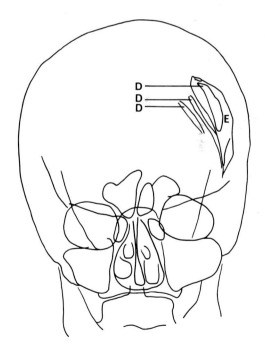

(b) *PA view.*
Double densities (D) are seen again
indicating bony overlap and the major
fragment (E) has a lower density than the
surrounding skull, indicating that it is lying
in a slightly different plane and is
depressed. Depressed skull fractures are
usually associated with significant brain
injury.

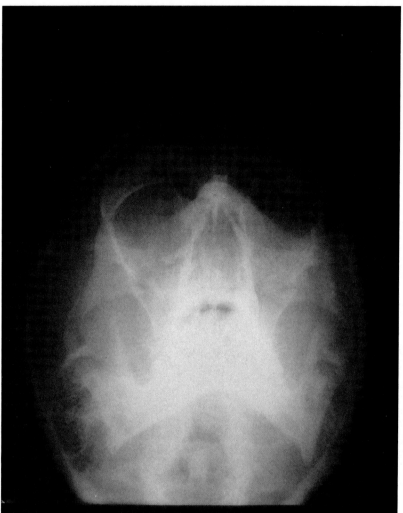

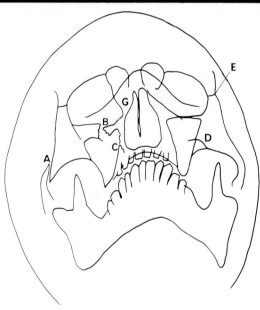

28   **Facial fracture.**
The zygoma, maxilla and orbital margin are mutually supportive. A fracture of one usually involves a fracture of at least one of the others. Facial fractures may be unilateral or bilateral and, in severe cases, the facial bones can be detached from the skull. Fracture of the inferior orbital margins leads to diplopia.

In this example, the fractures on the right side involve the zygomatic arch (A), inferior orbital margin (B) and medial wall of the maxillary antrum (C). On the left, there is a fracture running across the junction of the zygoma with the lateral wall of the maxillary antrum (D). A fracture may be accompanied by diastasis of the fronto-zygomatic sutures (E) but, in this case, it is intact. There is deformity of the nose (G) secondary to bony cartilaginous injury.

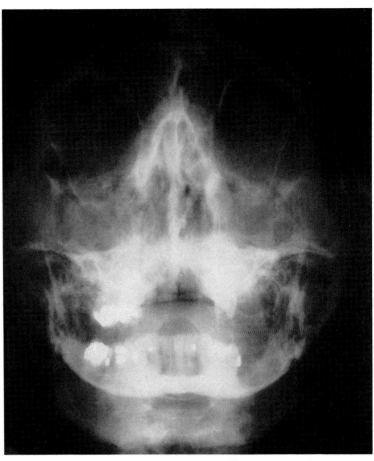

29   Central facial fracture.
This is a more severe injury which caused
depression of the central part of the face.
The depression is not evident on this view
but some of the associated fractures are.
They involve the medial walls of both
orbits and the frontal sinuses (A), both
inferior orbital margins (B), the left
zygoma (C) and the medial wall of the
right maxillary antrum (D).

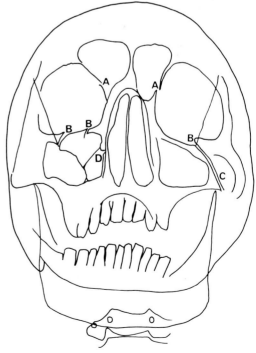

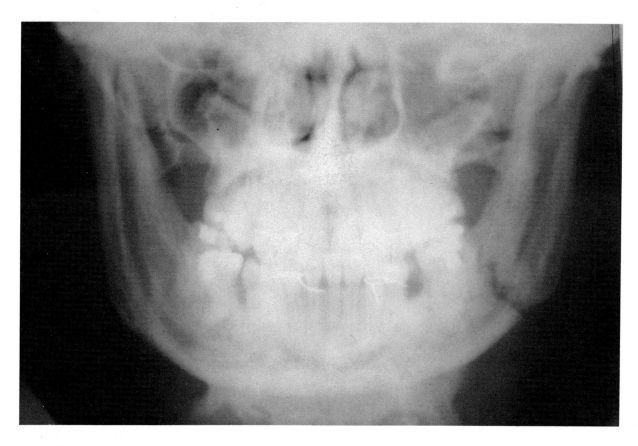

30 **Fracture of the mandible.**

(a) *AP view.*
There is a fracture of the angle of the mandible (A). In any ring structure such as the mandible, it is important to look for a balancing fracture on the other side. The opposite condyle is the usual site. No such fracture is present in this case.

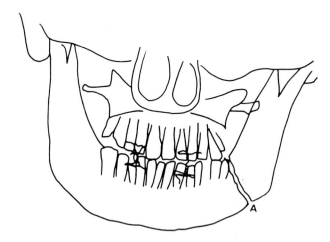

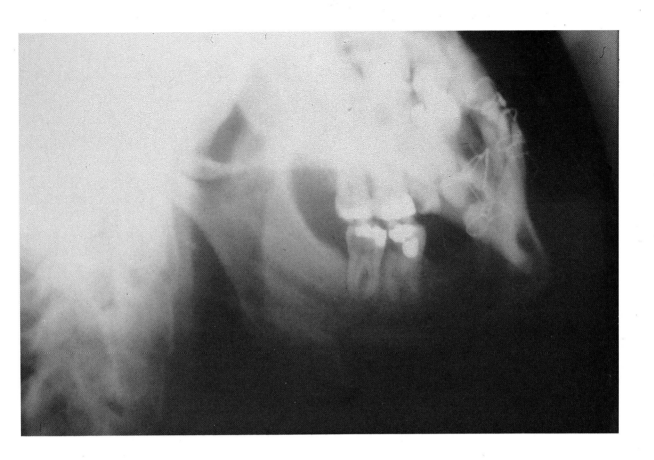

(b) *Oblique view.*
The branches of the fracture (A) communicate with the roots of the last two molars (B and C), a common situation. This makes the fracture compound. Another common site is at the root of the canine tooth. Dental wiring (D) is present to fix the jaw.

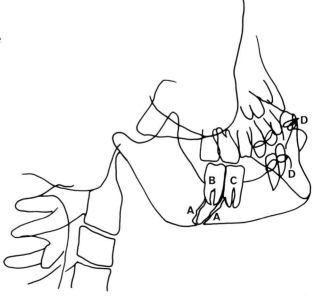

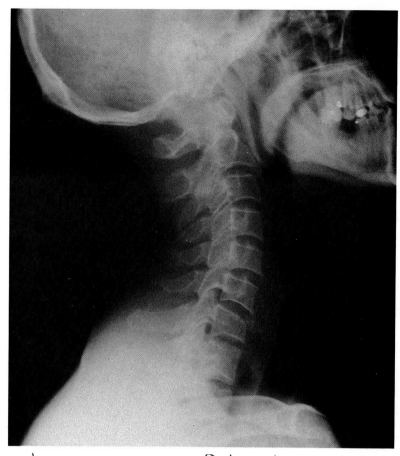

31 Spinal fractures.
Spinal fractures may
vary from minor and
self-limiting to those
which cause complete
transection of the cord.
In **31**, an avulsion
fracture of the antero-
superior margin of CV7
(A), the injury was
minor. However, even
when the bony injury
appears slight, sufficient
flexion may have
occurred at the time of
injury to produce cord
damage.

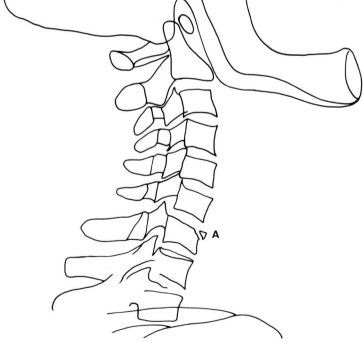

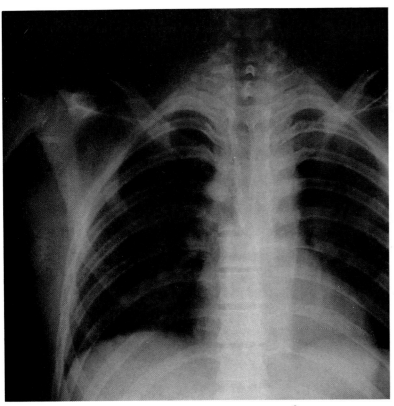

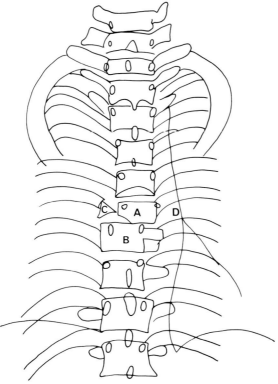

32 **Fracture dislocation of the thoracic spine.**

(a) *AP view.*

There is gross lateral dislocation of DV6 (A) on 7 (B). A small right infero-lateral fragment of DV6 (C) maintains its normal relationship with DV7. There is a paraspinal soft tissue shadow (D), the result of an associated haematoma.

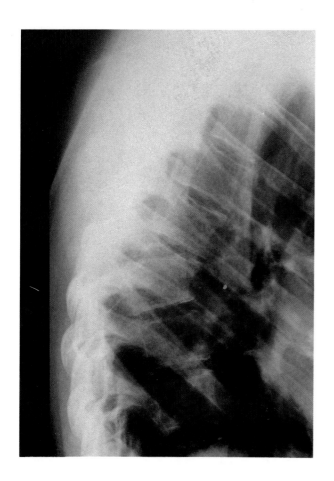

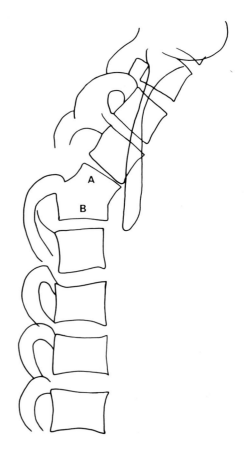

(b) *Lateral view.*
There is anterior wedging of DV6 (A) on 7 (B). The adjacent vertebral margins cannot be distinguished.

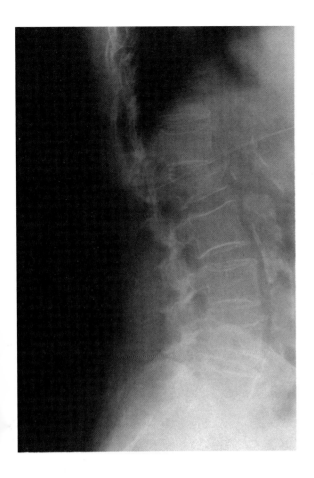

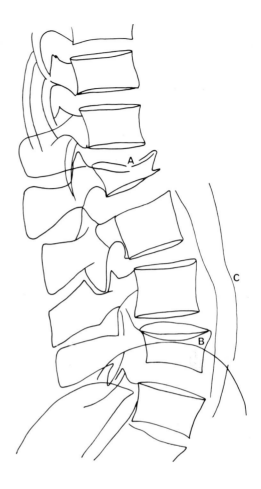

33 **Compression fractures of lumbar vertebral bodies.**

Fractures of the vertebral bodies are usually stable unless there is accompanying damage to the neural arch, apophyseal joints or supporting ligaments. They can occur after minor trauma, which may have passed unnoticed in elderly, osteoporotic patients.

(a) *Lateral view.*
There is compression of LV1 (A) and partial compression of LV4 (B). The bones look osteoporotic and the heavy aortic calcification (C) shows that this is an elderly patient.

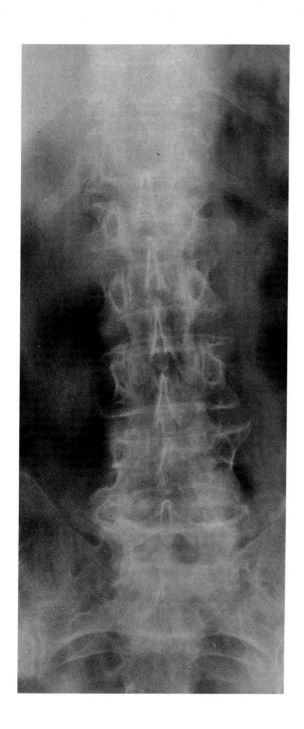
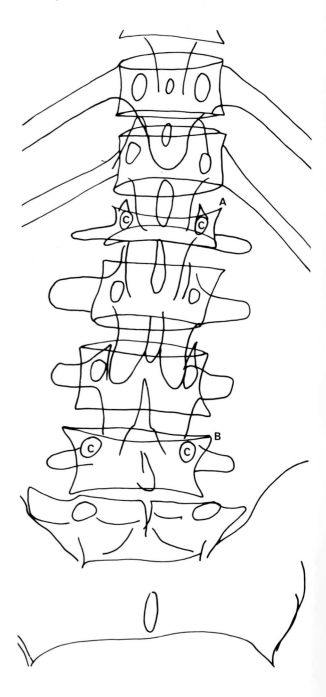

(b) *AP view.*
The LV1 fracture (A) can be seen clearly.
The LV4 fracture (B) is less obvious. The
pedicles (C) at both levels are intact,
making collapse secondary to bony
metastases unlikely.

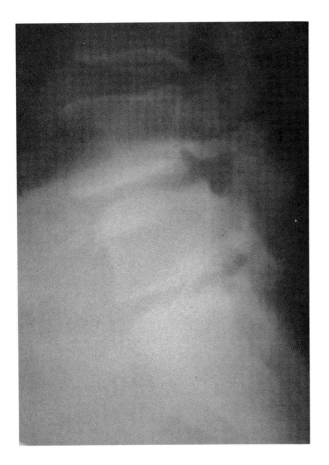
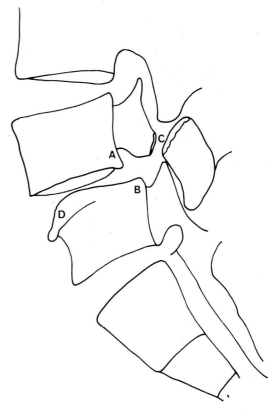

34 **Spondylolistheses.**

This is anterior displacement of one lumbar vertebral body on another or of LV5 on S1. It is only rarely due to acute trauma and is more commonly related to stress injury of the pars articularis or abnormalities of the facet joints.

As in this example, the forward slip is best seen on the lateral view. L4 is displaced anteriorly on L5, the loss of alignment being most clearly seen at the posterior aspects of the vertebral bodies (A and B). The defect in the pars interarticularis of L4 (C) is clearly seen. The sclerosis of the margins of the defect and the antero-superior L5 osteophyte (D) indicate that the abnormality has been present for some time.

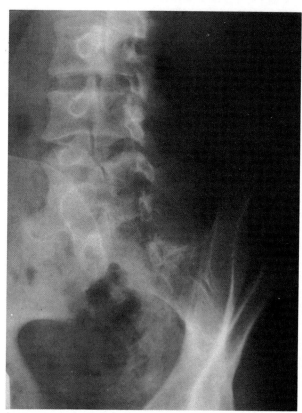

35   Spondylolisthesis of L5 on S1 in a different patient.
The articular facets and pars interarticularis are more clearly seen in an oblique view. Their appearance has been likened to a 'Scottie dog'. The normal appearance is best seen at L4. The nose of the dog is the transverse process (A), the ear the superior articular facet (B), the eye the pedicle (C), the neck the pars interarticularis (D) and the foreleg the inferior articular facet (E). The defect in spondylolisthesis is a break in the neck, seen at L5 (F).

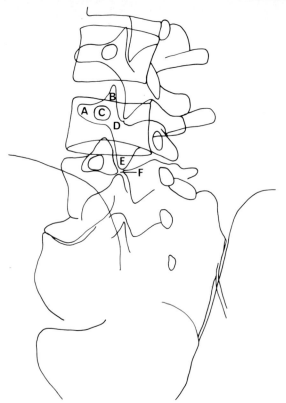

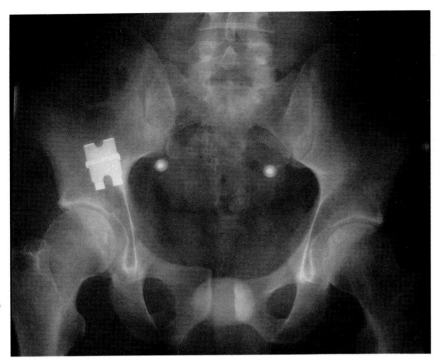

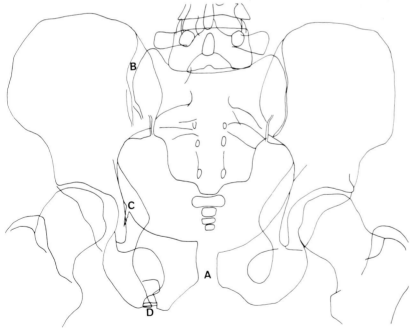

36 **Pelvic fractures and dislocation.**
As mentioned under mandibular fractures, when a fracture occurs in one part of a ring structure, it is important to look for a balancing fracture or dislocation elsewhere. The pelvic dislocations and fractures in this patient illustrate the point in two places.

There are dislocations of the pubic symphysis (A) and the right sacro-iliac joint (B) which is wider than the left. There are also fractures on both sides of the right obdurator foramen, involving both the superior (C) and inferior (D) pubic rami.

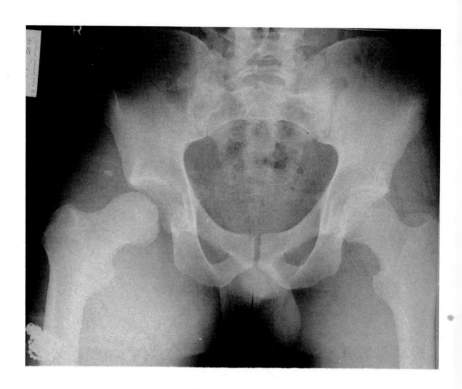

37   **Dislocation of the right hip.**
This is a posterior dislocation which is more common than anterior dislocation. The femoral head (A) is displaced postero-superiorly from the acetabular cavity (B).

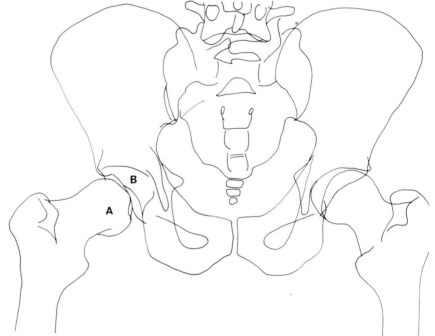

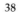

38

Fractured neck of femur.
Fractures of the femoral neck are common in the elderly and are often related to osteoporosis. Femoral neck fractures may be intra or extra-capsular. Those which are in the anatomical neck of the femur are intracapsular. As most of the blood supply to the femoral head comes from small epiphyseal vessels easily damaged by a femoral neck fracture, intracapsular fractures are frequently complicated by avascular necrosis of the femoral head. This example shows an intracapsular fracture (A) of the right femoral neck.

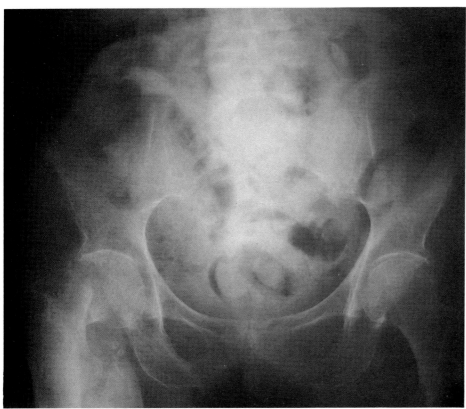

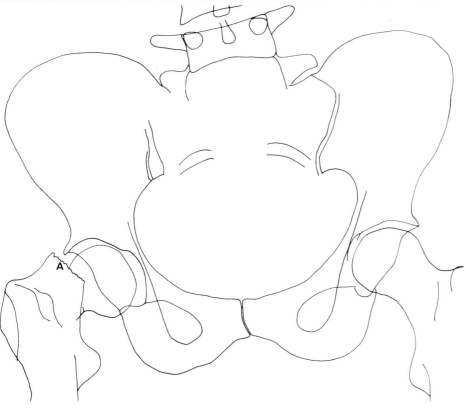

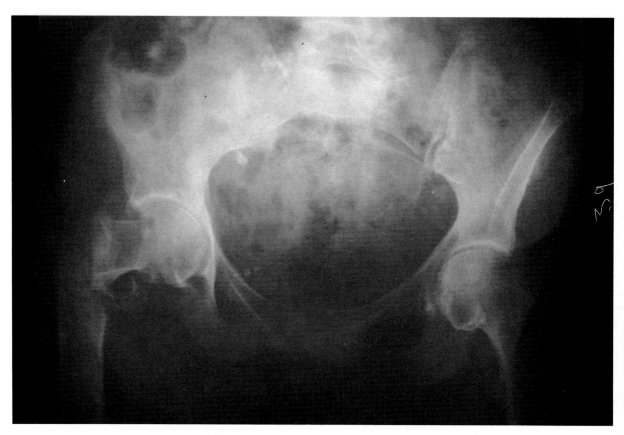

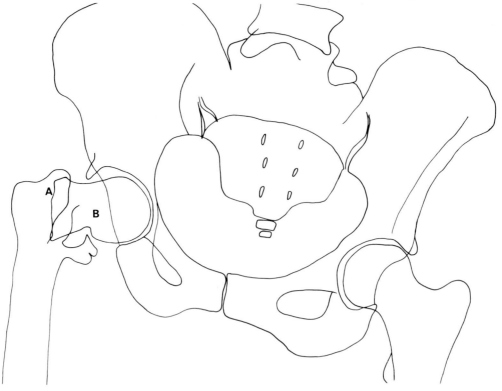

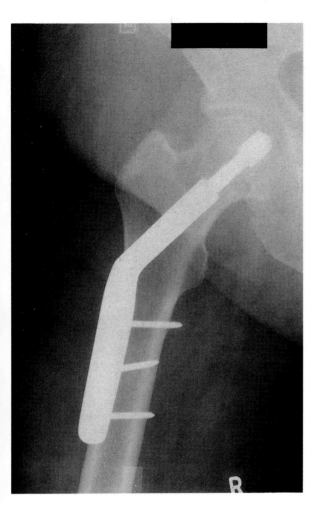

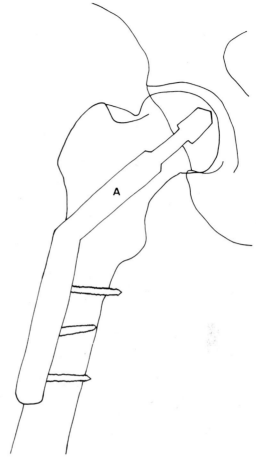

40   **Reduced femoral neck fracture in a different patient.**
There is internal fixation using a three-hole Zimmer nail plate (A). The fracture line is not clearly seen. Internal fixation speeds healing and avoids long-term immobility in traction.

39   **Intertrochanteric fracture of the right femur.**
◄   As mentioned above, this is an extracapsular fracture and is much less likely to be complicated by avascular necrosis. There is a fracture line (Á) running across the intertrochanteric region. There is an associated varus deformity of the femoral neck (B).

41 **Slipped proximal femoral epiphysis. Early appearances.**
This is probably an example of a stress injury. It occurs in adolescents, more often boys and more frequently in overweight individuals. It is bilateral in approximately one third of cases, which means that there is not always a normal opposite side for comparison.

(a) *AP view.*
In this case, the AP view looks virtually normal which may occur if the displacement is posterior.
Features to look for in the AP view are:
i)   displacement of the medial third of the metaphysis from the acetabulum,
ii) a line drawn along the lateral aspect of the femoral neck and extended proximally does not include the lateral part of the femoral head,
iii) there may be a widened epiphyseal plate.
None of these features is present in this case.

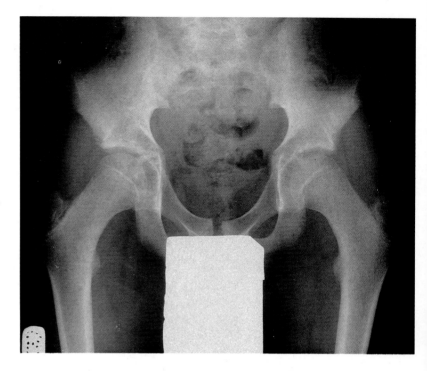

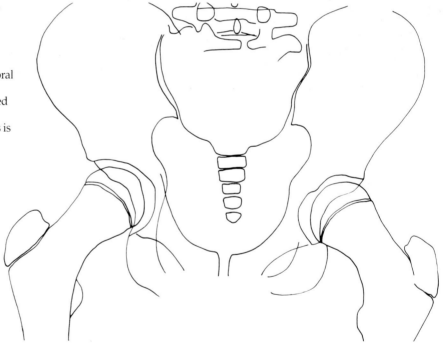

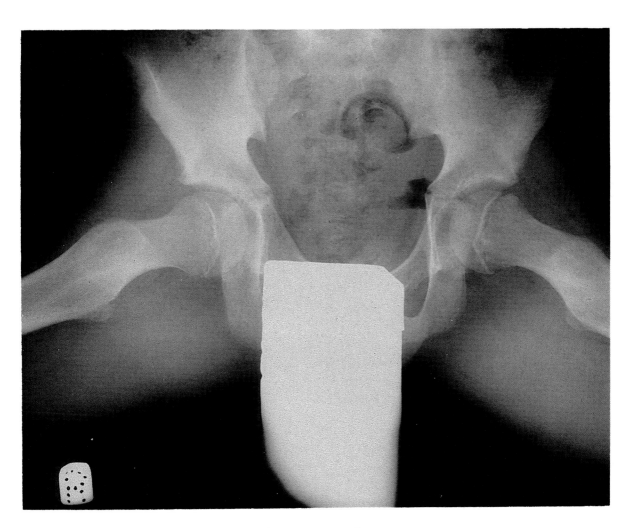

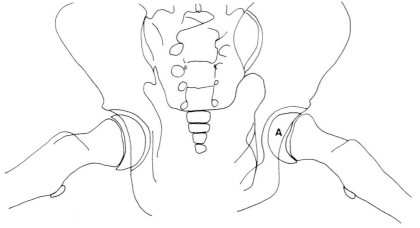

(b) *Lateral view.*
    The left femoral
    epiphysis (A) can be seen
    tilted posteriorly. A
    lateral view should
    always be taken because,
    as in this case, it may
    show the abnormality
    when the AP view is
    apparently normal.

61

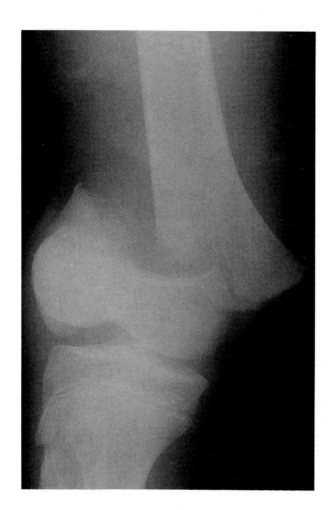
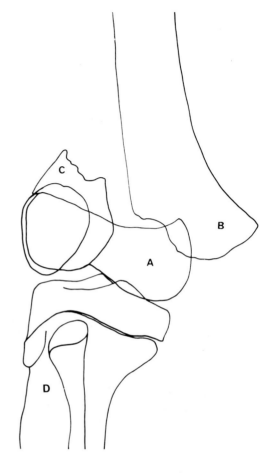

42   **Fracture and dislocation of the distal femoral epiphysis and metaphysis.**

(a)   *AP view.*
The epiphysis (A) is almost completely separated from the metaphysis (B). A lateral fragment of the metaphysis (C) remains attached to the epiphysis. As well as postero-lateral dislocation, there is also a considerable rotational deformity as the tibia and fibula (D) are seen in a virtually lateral position.

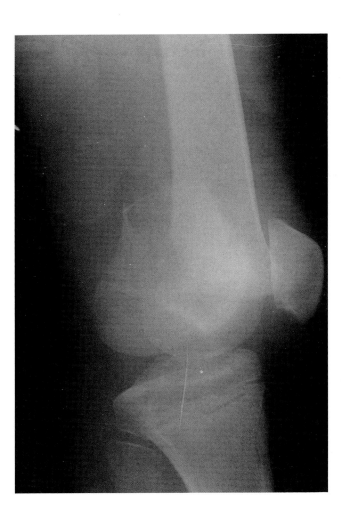
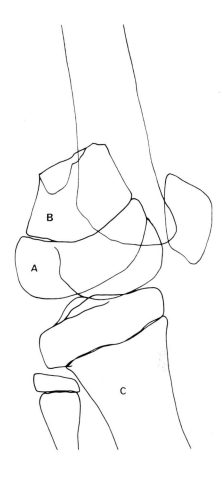

(b) *Lateral view.*
The posterior displacement of the epiphysis (A) and its metaphyseal fragment (B) is clearly seen. The proximal tibia and fibula (C) are in a very oblique (virtually AP) position, confirming the rotational deformity. Fractures and dislocations involving the epiphyseal plate may interfere with subsequent growth.

63

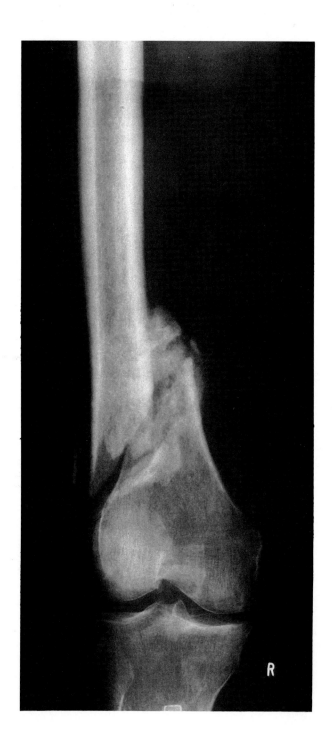

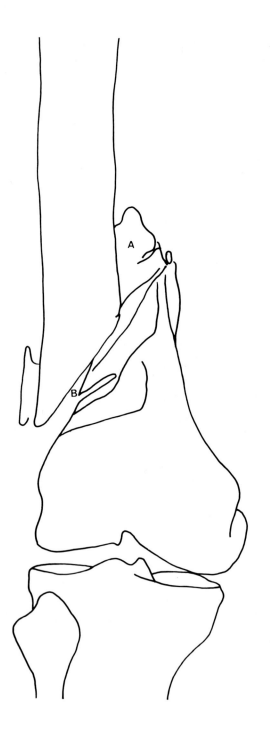

43   Healing fracture of the distal femur.

    (a)   *AP view.*

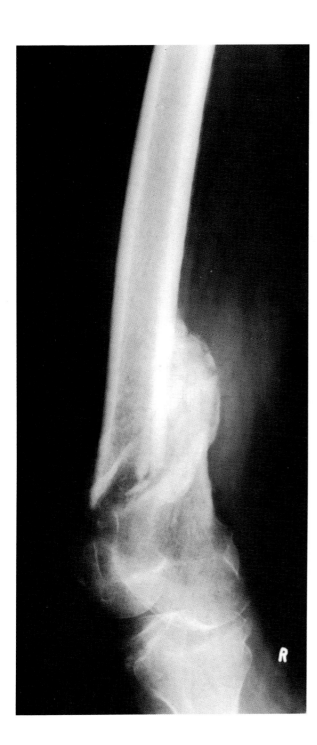

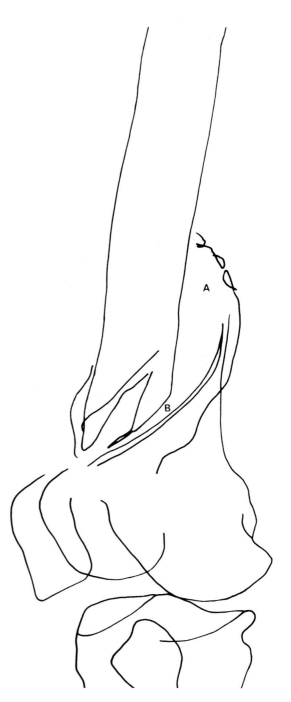

(b) *Oblique view.*
Both views show good callus formation (A)
across the fracture site. This indicates that
union is taking place, although the fracture
line (B) is still seen clearly.

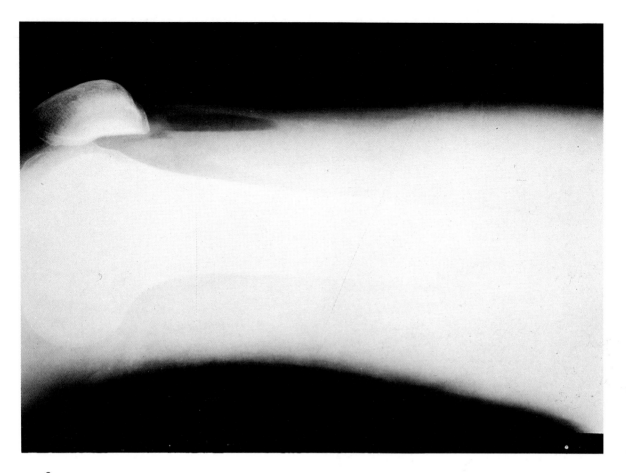

a

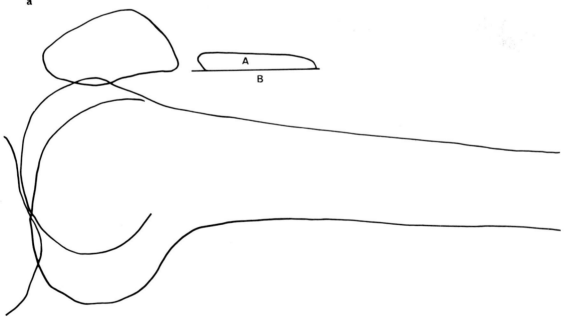

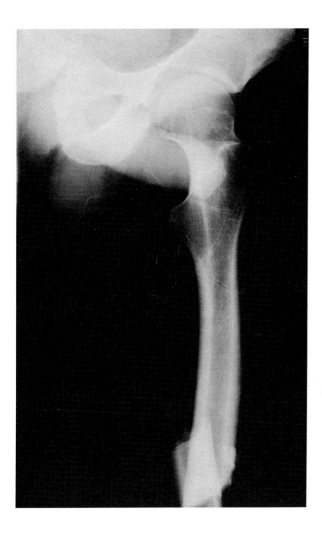

 b

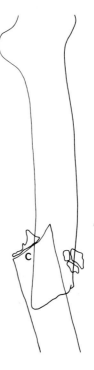

44   Fat/fluid level in the suprapatellar pouch.

(a)   Supine lateral film.
There is a distinct level between the
radiolucent fat (A) and the fluid below (B).
This is only seen when a horizontal x-ray
beam, tangential to the fluid level, is used.
The fat comes from bone marrow. The fluid is
blood. Such an appearance indicates an
underlying fracture, usually around the knee.

(b)   Femoral shaft of the same patient.
In this case, rather unusually, the fracture is
in the mid-femoral shaft (C).

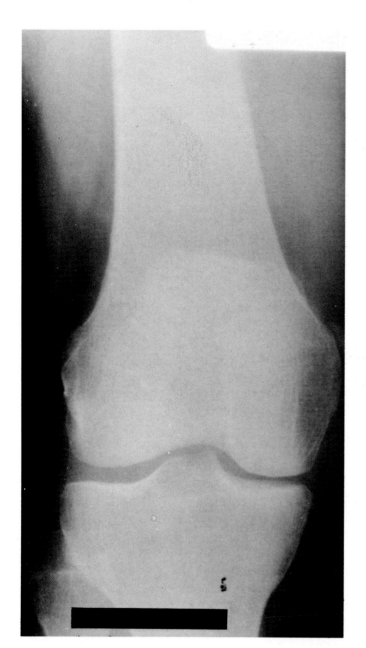

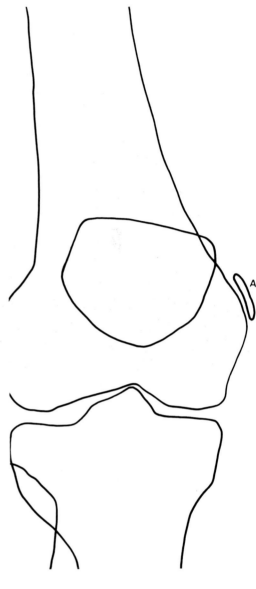

45 **Pellegrini-Stieda lesion.**
There is soft tissue calcification (A) medial to
the medial femoral condyle. This is probably
the result of chronic trauma and occurs, for
instance, in horse riders.

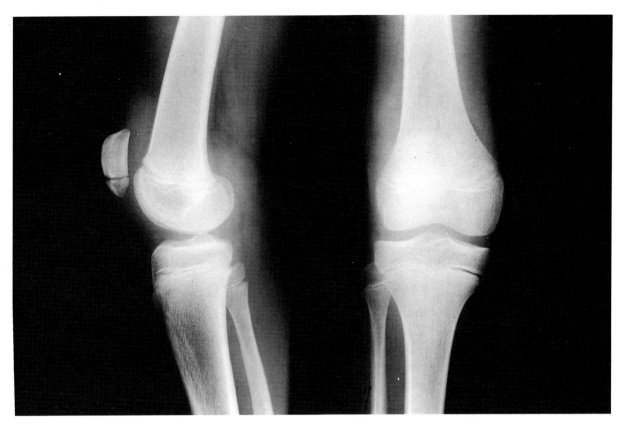

46 **Fracture of the lower pole of the patella.**

(a) *Lateral view.*
On the lateral view, the clear-cut relatively horizontal line (A) differentiates this from a congenital bipartite patella.

(b) *AP view.*
The fracture is not seen as it is obscured by the epiphyseal plate.

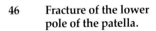
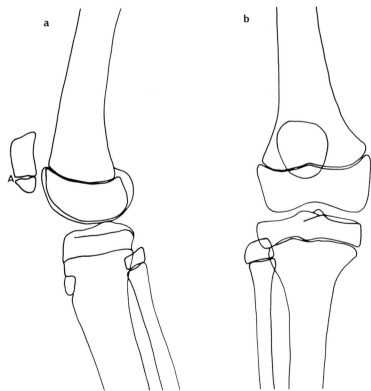

a

b

69

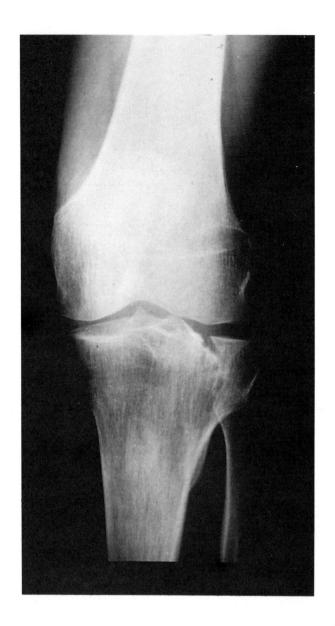

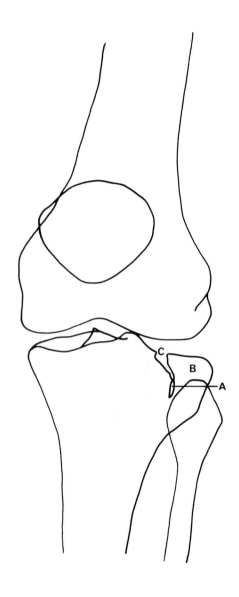

47   Fracture of the lateral tibial condyle.

(a) *AP view.*
There is a vertical fracture (A) separating the
lateral part of the tibial plateau (B) and
communicating with the knee joint (C).

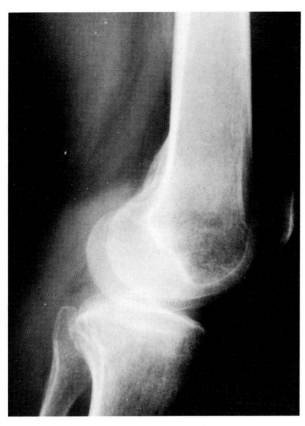

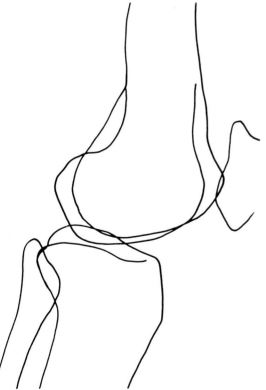

(b) *Lateral view.*
     The fracture cannot be seen. This illustrates
     the need, mentioned elsewhere in the text,
     for two views of a joint at right angles to each
     other.

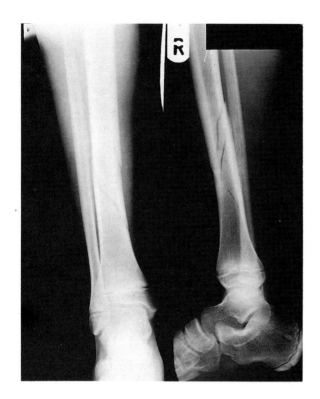
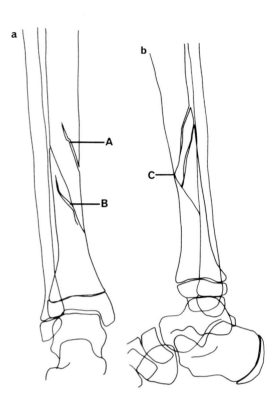

48   **Spiral fracture of the distal third of the tibia.**

(a)   *AP view.*

(b)   *Lateral view.*
        The apparently separate fracture lines (A and
        B) on the AP view (a) are seen to join with
        each other anteriorly (C) on the lateral view
        (b). This is a continuous spiral fracture rather
        than separate fractures. It allows a greater
        surface area for healing than a transverse
        fracture and so union is likely to be more
        rapid.

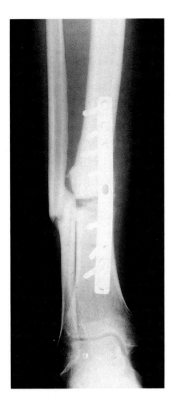
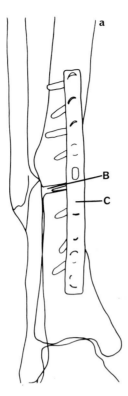

49   Fractures of the distal thirds of the tibia and fibula.

(a)   AP view.

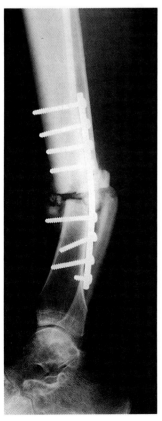
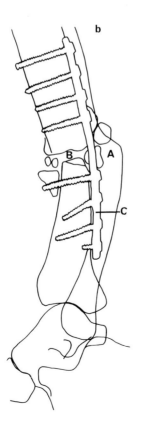

(b)   Lateral view.
The fibular fracture has healed with deformity (A). There is non-union of the tibial fracture (B). This may be due to interposition of soft tissues between the bone ends or to excessive distraction of the fragments. The oval holes in the fixing nail plates (C) are designed to let the fracture ends impact and prevent this happening. The union of the fibula is also helping to keep the ends apart.

50   Stress fracture of the upper tibial shaft.
Repeated minor trauma may tend to stress fractures. Athletes, ballet dancers and parachutists among others are prone to such lesions.
The upper tibia is a recognised site for a stress fracture.

(a)   AP view.

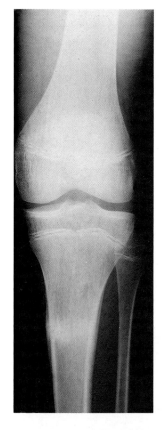
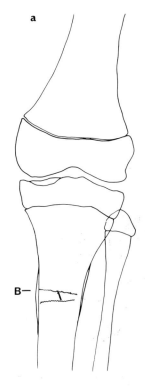

(b)   Lateral view.
In both views there is a sclerotic band (A) in the upper tibia with an associated periosteal reaction (B). No fracture line is visible as is frequently the case.
It is important to recognise stress fractures for what they are, since radiologically and pathologically they can be confused with neoplasms. Follow-up films after a few weeks' rest are often helpful in the differential diagnosis as stress fractures should heal eventually.

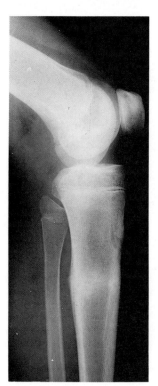
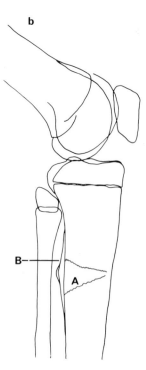

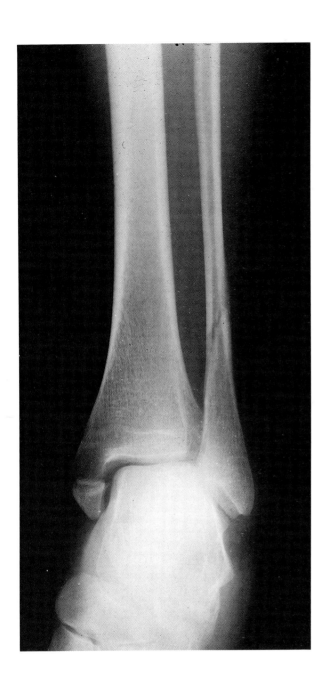

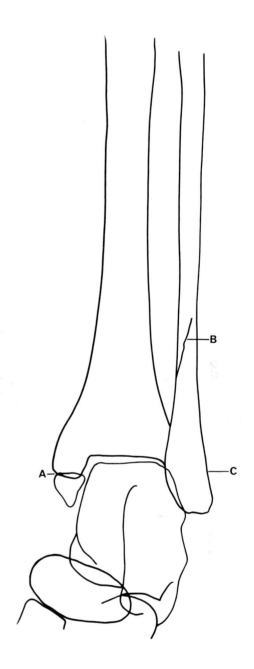

51   **Pott's fracture of the ankle.**

(a)   *AP view.*
      There are fractures of the medial malleolus
      (A) of the tibia and of the distal fibula (B)
      above the lateral malleolus (C). The head of
      the talus is slightly displaced laterally
      (arrowed) showing that the fracture is
      unstable. The stability of the ankle depends
      on the integrity of the malleoli and the
      supporting ligaments.

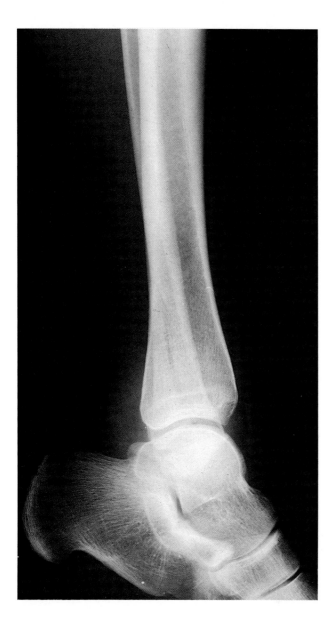

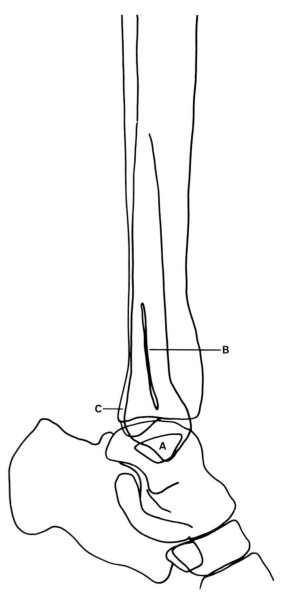

(b) *Lateral view.*
     The separate distal fragment of the medial
     malleolus (A) is difficult to see due to bony
     overlap. The fibular fracture (B) is seen
     clearly. The third malleolus, the posterior
     aspect of the distal tibia (C) is intact.

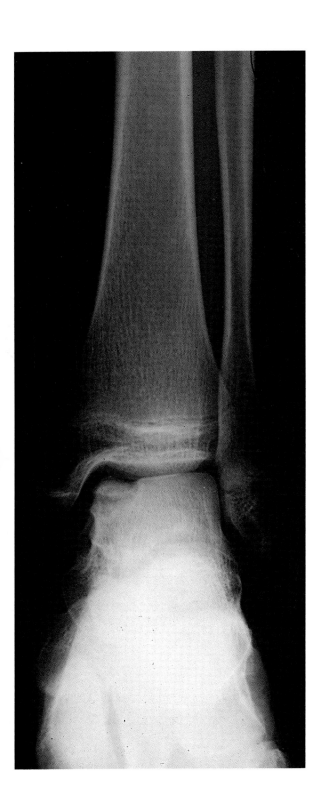

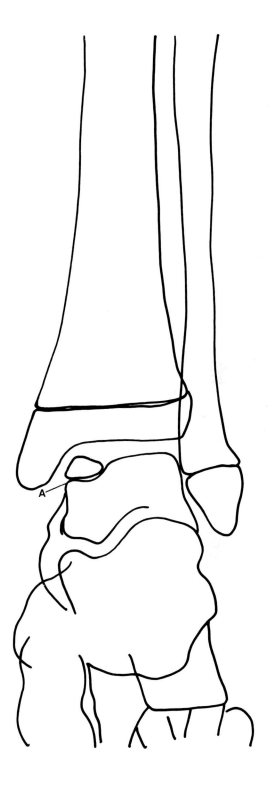

52 **Fracture of talus.**
There is a fracture (A) of the medial aspect of
the proximal articular surface of the talus.

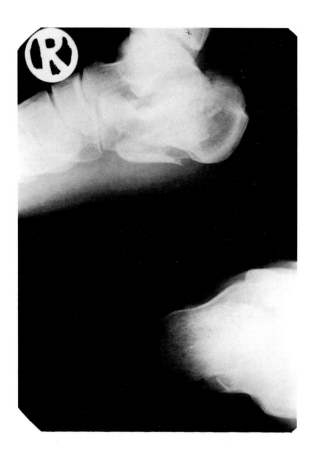

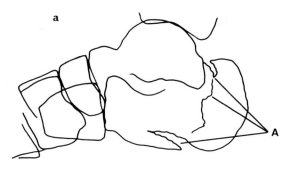

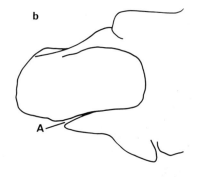

53   Fracture of calcaneus.
Calcaneal fractures are usually caused by the patient falling from a height and landing on his feet.

(a)   *Lateral view.*
In the lateral view, the calcaneus is flattened and the irregular fracture (A) is seen clearly.

(b)   *Axial view.*
The axial view also shows the fracture (A). If a fracture is suspected clinically but not seen, Bohler's angle should be measured (see diagram). The acute angle should be 28–40 degrees. An angle of less than 28 degrees indicates a probable fracture.

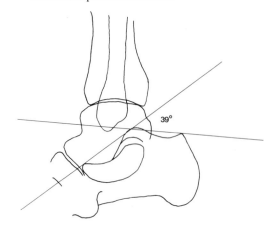

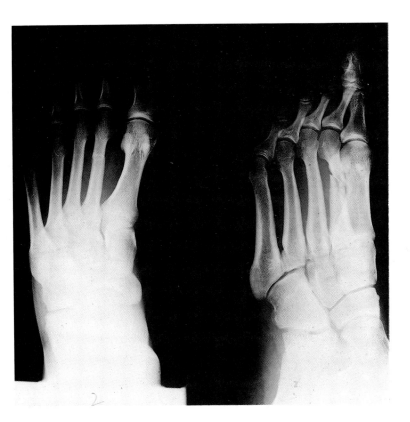

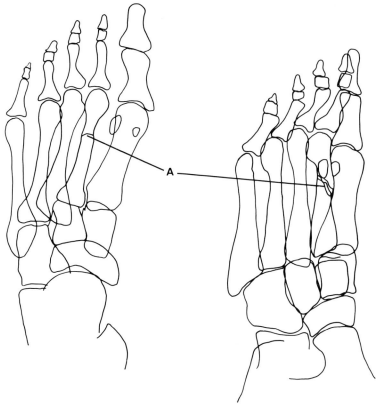

54   Fracture of the second
      metatarsal (A).

79

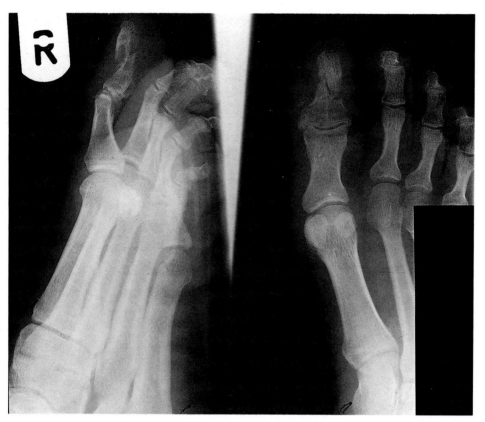

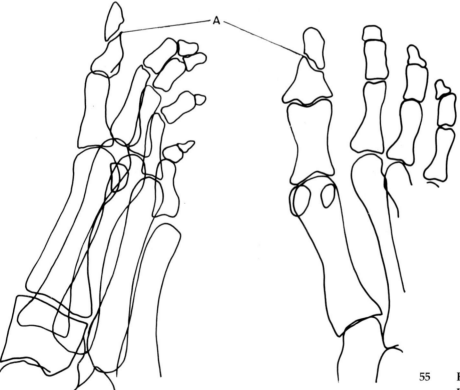

55   Fracture of the first terminal phalanx (A).

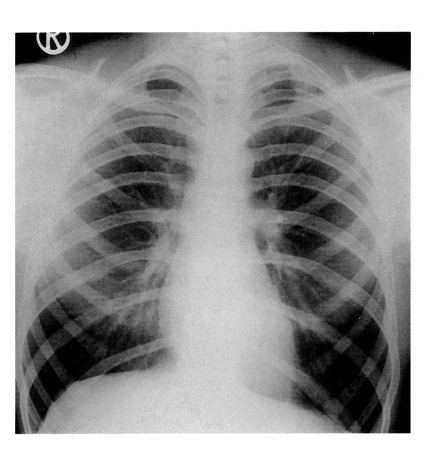

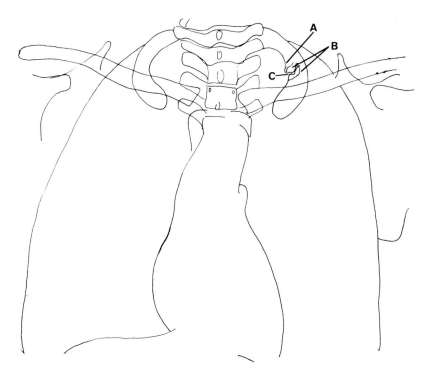

56 **Fracture of the left first rib.**
A stress fracture in this site may be caused by carrying a heavy pack. There is slight expansion (A) of the anterior aspect of the first rib. There is a little sclerosis (B) on both sides of the fracture line (C).

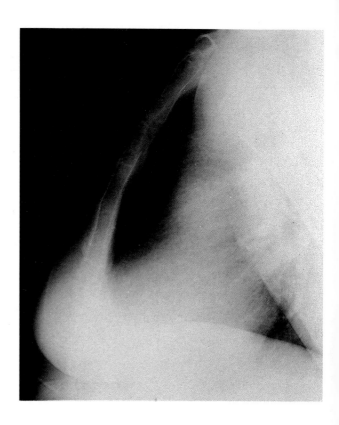

57 **Fractured sternum. Lateral view.**
Do not mistake the normal manubrio-sternal
joint (A) for a fracture. The fracture (B) is
below the joint and is causing discontinuity in
the anterior and posterior sternal margins.

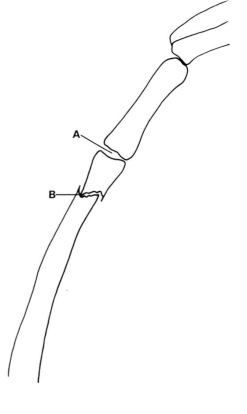

82

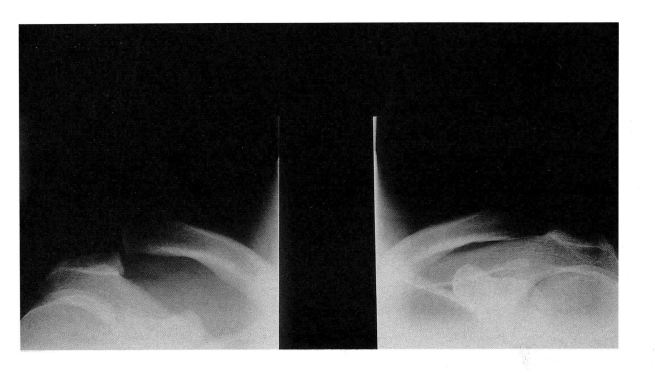

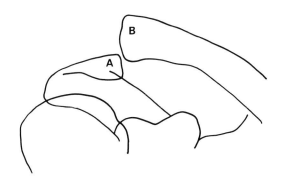
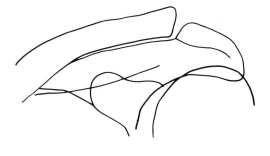

58   **Dislocation of the right acromio-clavicular joint.**
The acromion (A) is depressed with respect to the distal clavicle (B). The normal left side is shown for comparison.

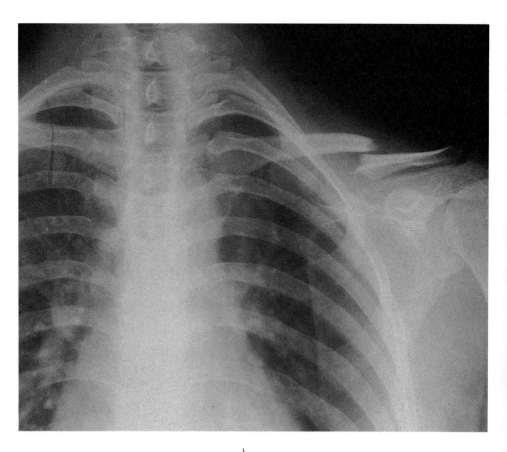

59   Fracture of the left clavicle.
Such fractures are common and easily
recognised. The fracture (A) is seen clearly.
There is overlap of the bone ends.

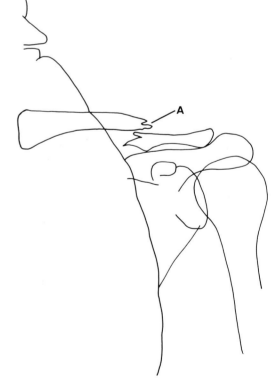

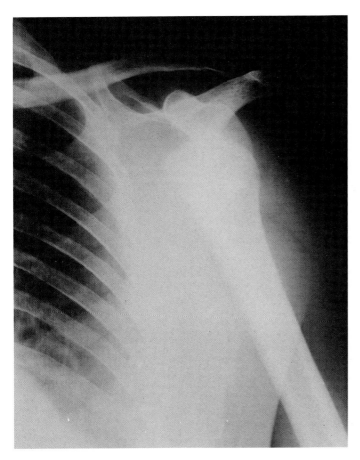

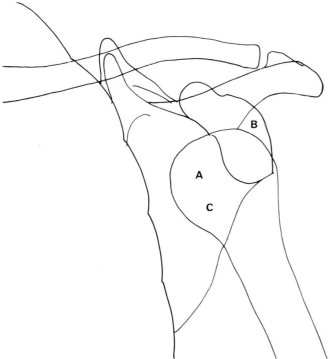

60   **Anterior dislocation of the shoulder.**
This is the common form of shoulder
dislocation. The humeral head (A) is
displaced antero-medially from the glenoid
fossa (B) and is superimposed on the scapula
(C).

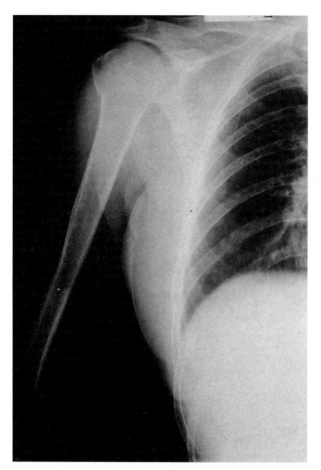

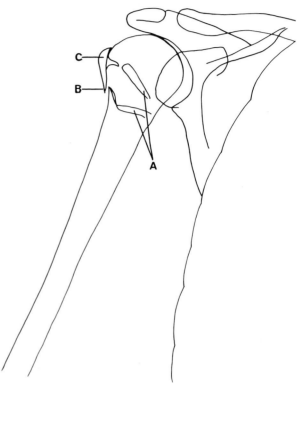

61 **Fracture of the humeral neck with avulsion of the greater tuberosity.**
The overlapping margins of the humeral neck fracture can be seen as double densities running more or less transversely (A). There is a fracture line (B) running across the base of the greater tuberosity (C).

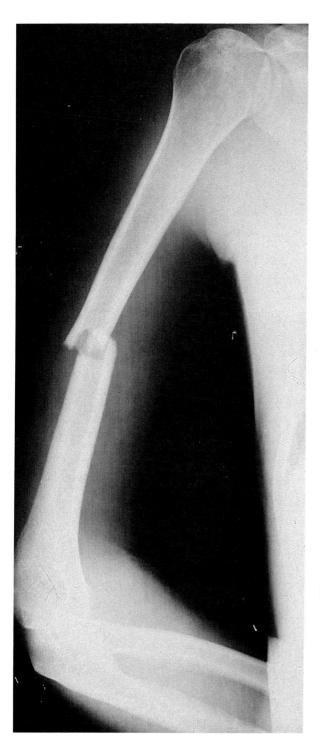
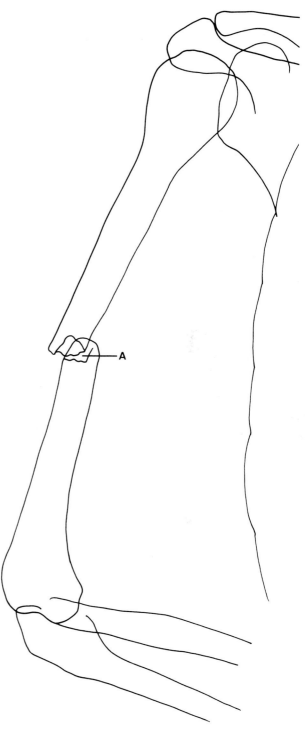

62   **Fracture of the shaft of the humerus.**
The transverse humeral shaft fracture is seen
clearly (A).

87

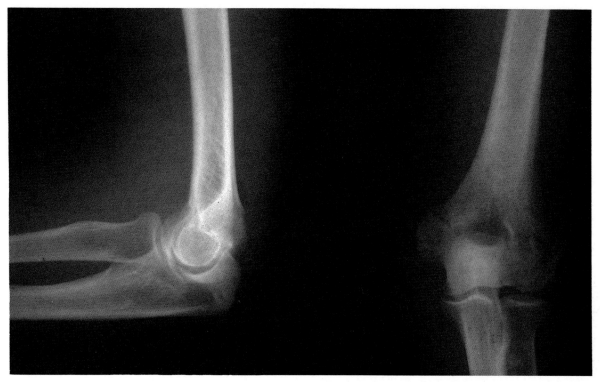

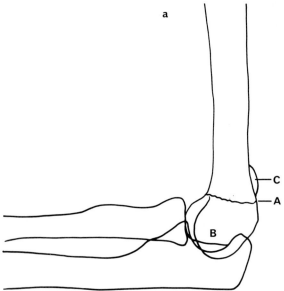

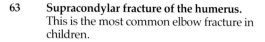

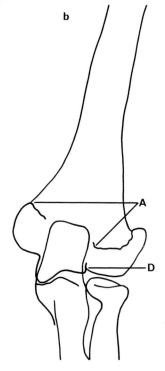

63   **Supracondylar fracture of the humerus.**
This is the most common elbow fracture in children.

(a)   *Lateral view.*
The fracture line (A) runs across the humerus above the condyles (B). There is displacement of the radiolucent fat pad (C) from the olecranon fossa. This indicates effusion into the joint and an underlying fracture, even if the fracture line is invisible.

(b)   *AP view.*
In addition to the transverse supracondylar fracture line (A), there is a vertical intercondylar fracture (D) extending from the supracondylar fracture into the elbow joint.

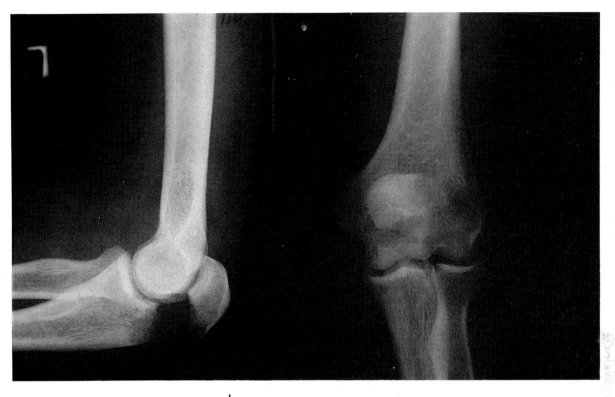

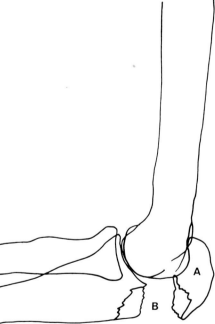

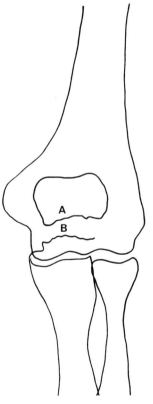

64 Fracture of the olecranon.
The olecranon (A) is separated from the rest
of the ulna by a wide fracture (B)
communicating with the elbow joint. The
fracture is less clearly seen on the AP view.

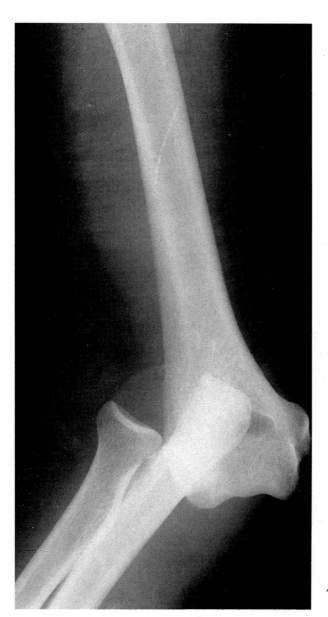

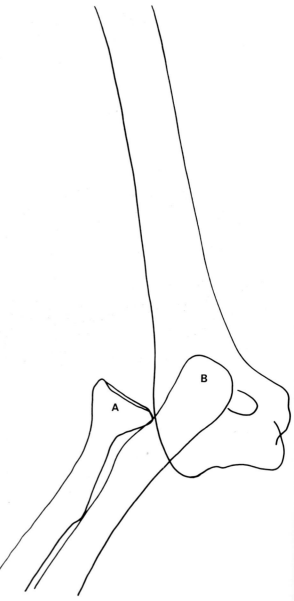

65 **Elbow dislocation.**
There is anterior dislocation of the head of the radius (A) and the olecranon of the ulna (B) with respect to the humerus. This type of dislocation is less common than posterior dislocation of the elbow.

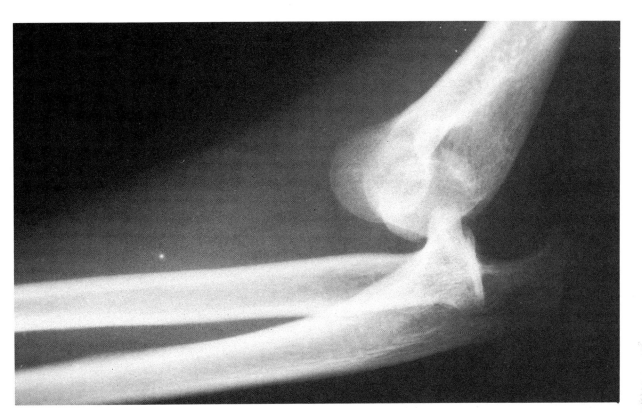

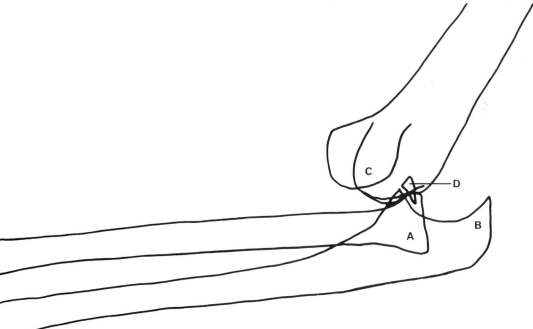

66   Posterior dislocation of the elbow.
This is a more common injury. There is
posterior dislocation of the head of the radius
(A) and olecranon (B) with respect to the
distal humerus (C). The coronoid process of
the ulna (D) is avulsed, a common
accompaniment.

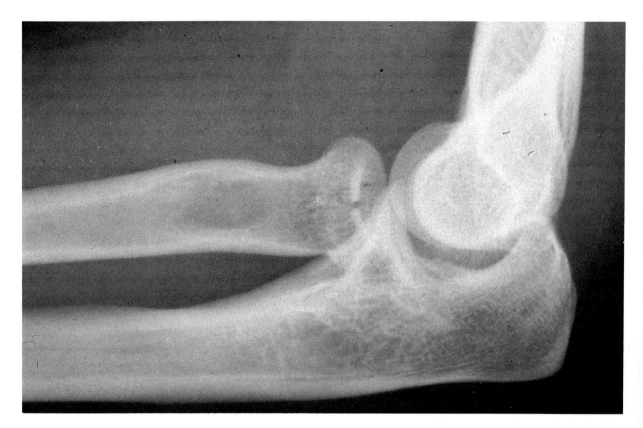

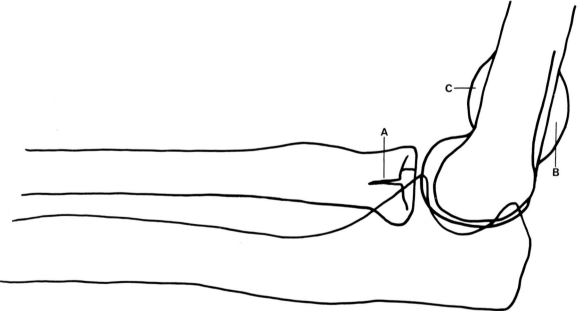

67 **Fracture of the radial head.**
The fracture line (A) extends to the articular surface. Displacement is minimal and such fractures can be missed.
As mentioned in **63**, fat pad displacement is an important indicator of fracture. Both the posterior (B) and anterior fat pads (C) are faintly seen and are displaced.

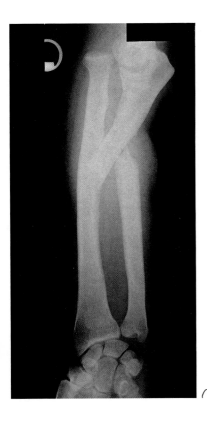

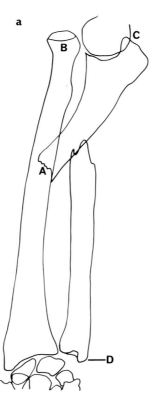

68   **Monteggia fracture/
      dislocation of the
      forearm.**
      Usually the radius and
      ulna both fracture
      together. If the ulna
      alone fractures and
      there is any
      foreshortening, the
      radial head dislocates.

(a)   *AP view of the forearm.*
      There is a fracture of the
      ulna (A) and the radial
      head (B) is dislocated.
      There must also be
      rotational deformity
      since the elbow (C) is
      seen in a lateral
      projection and the wrist
      (D) in an AP projection.

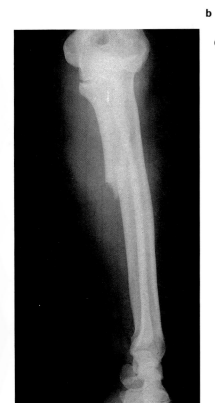

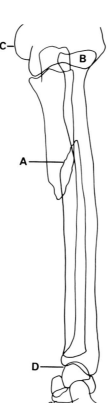

(b)   *Lateral view of forearm.*
      The ulnar fracture (A) is
      seen but the radial
      dislocation (B) is
      superimposed on the
      distal humerus. This
      time, the elbow (C), is
      seen in an AP projection
      and the wrist (D) in a
      lateral, confirming the
      90 degree rotation.

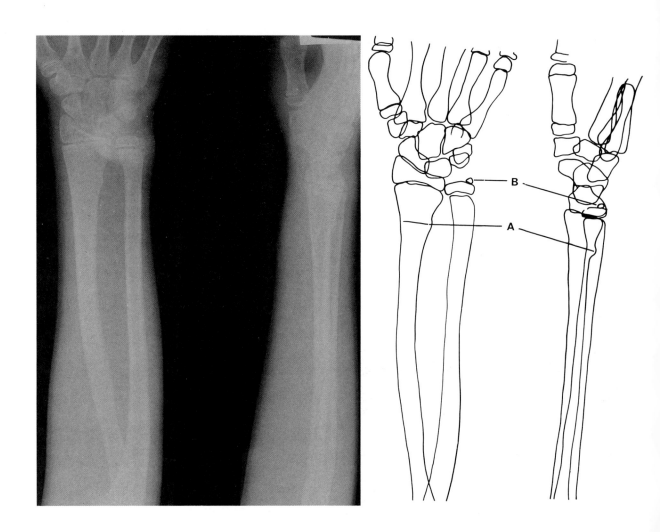

69 **'Greenstick' fracture of the radius.**
This type of fracture occurs in children.
Although a complete break is present, all
that may be seen radiographically is slight
buckling of the cortex. In this example,
there is slight buckling of the distal radial
cortex (A) and avulsion of the ulnar styloid
(B).

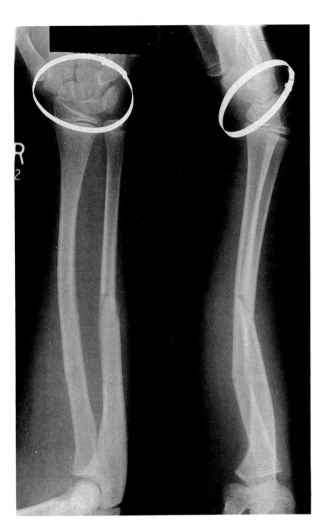

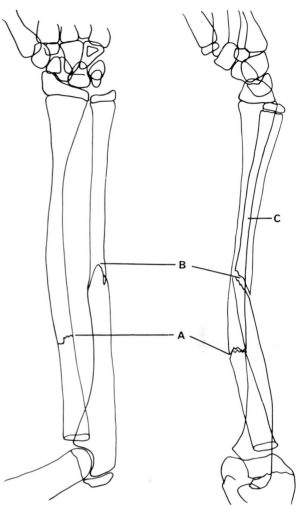

70   Fractures of the radius and ulna.
Complete fractures of the shafts of both
radius (A) and ulna (B) are present. There is
moderate posterior angulation of the distal
fragments (C).

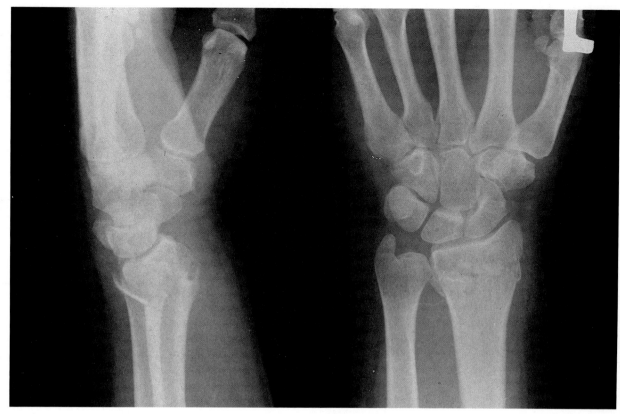

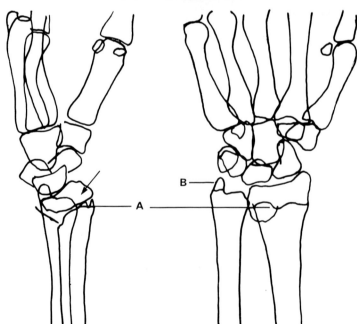

71   Colles' fracture of the wrist.
This is the commonest type of wrist
fracture, caused by the patient falling on an
outstretched hand. On physical
examination, the wrist has a characteristic

dinner-fork' deformity. On the radiograph,
there is a fracture of the distal radius (A)
with posterior tilting of the distal fragment
(arrowed). The ulnar styloid is avulsed (B).

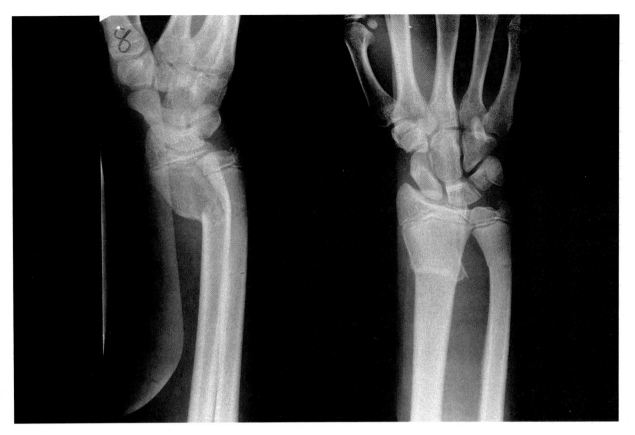

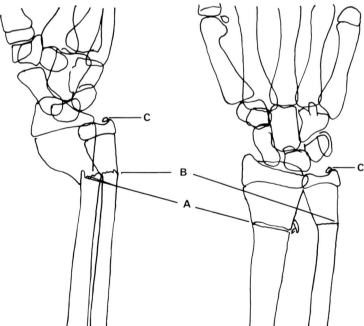

72 Smith's fracture of the wrist.
This is much rarer than a Colles' fracture. There are fractures of the distal radius (A) and ulna (B) with anterior angulation (arrowed). The ulnar styloid (C) is avulsed.

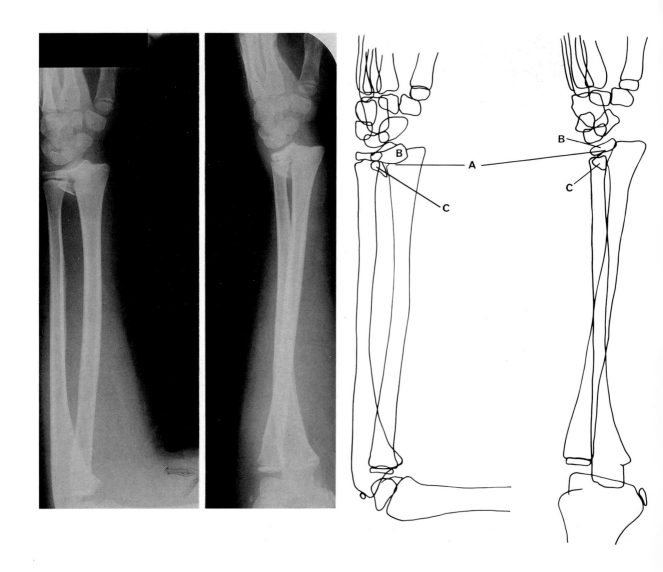

73   **Posterior displacement of the distal radial
epiphysis with an associated metaphyseal
fracture.**
As mentioned in **42**, fractures involving the
epiphyseal plate in children can interfere
with epiphyseal growth. There is a fracture
through the distal epiphyseal plate (A) and
the epiphysis (B) is displaced backwards. A
posterior fragment of metaphysis (C) has
been avulsed and remains attached to the
epiphysis.

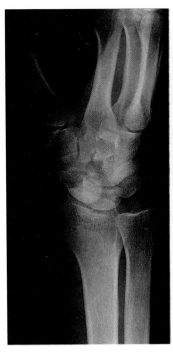
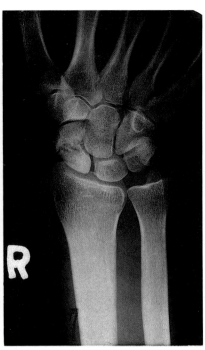

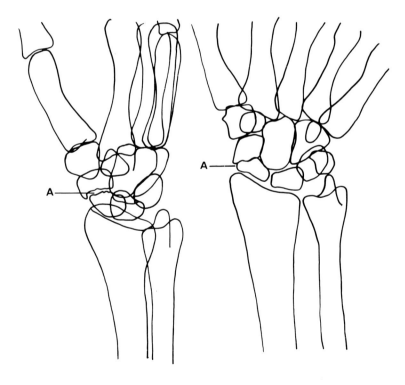

74   **Fracture of the scaphoid.**
The nutrient artery to the scaphoid enters its distal end. If the waist of the scaphoid is fractured, the proximal pole is, therefore, at risk of avascular necrosis. It is important to immobilise scaphoid fractures on clinical grounds even if the fracture line is not visible on the initial radiograph.

In this example, the fracture (A) through the waist of the scaphoid can be seen clearly on both the PA and oblique views.

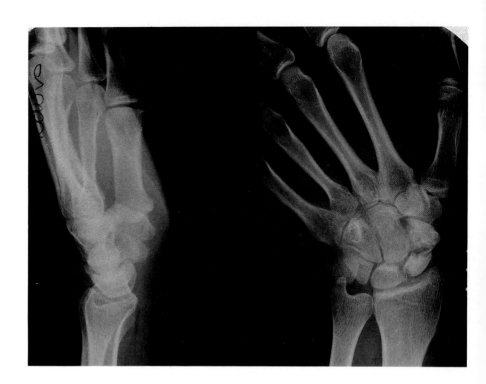

75   Avascular necrosis of the proximal pole of the scaphoid following fracture.
The fracture (A) has not united and can be seen clearly on the PA view. The density of the proximal pole (B) is increased, a sign of avascular necrosis. The abnormality is not clearly seen on the lateral view.

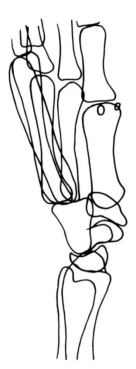 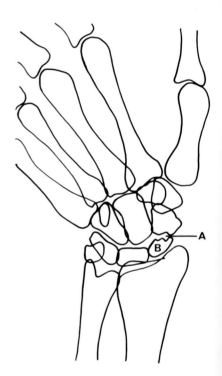

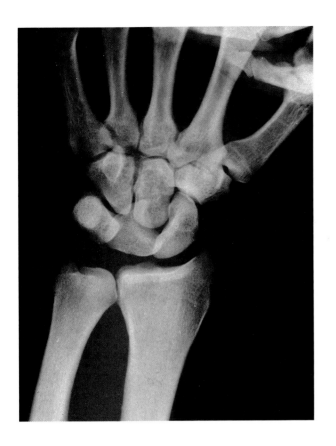

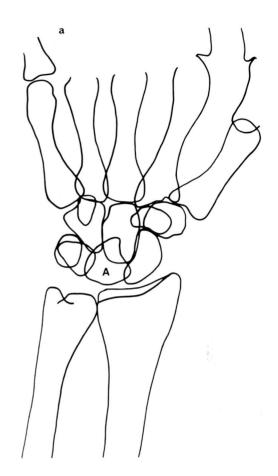

a

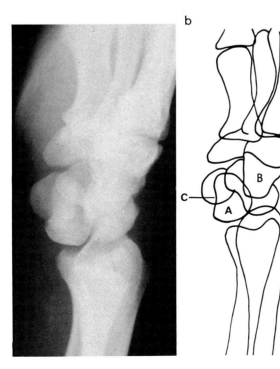

b

76   **Anterior dislocation of the lunate.**

(a)   *AP view.*
      The abnormality is difficult to see. The clue to
      the dislocation is the triangular shape of the
      lunate (A). It normally has a semilunar shape
      in this projection.

(b)   *Lateral view.*
      The dislocation is seen clearly. The lunate (A)
      is anterior to the rest of the carpus (B). It has
      been rotated through 90 degrees and its
      concave surface (C) is anterior.

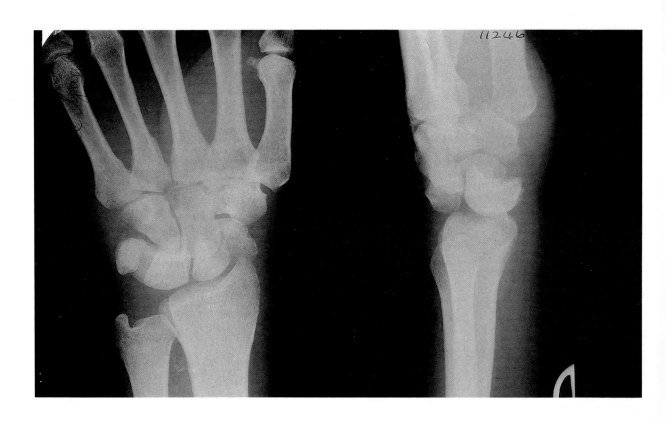

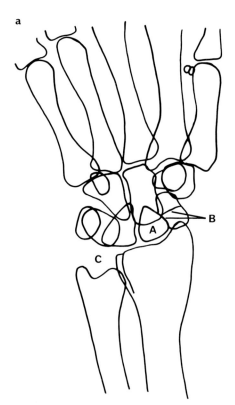

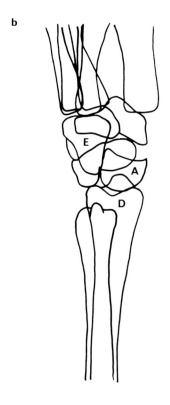

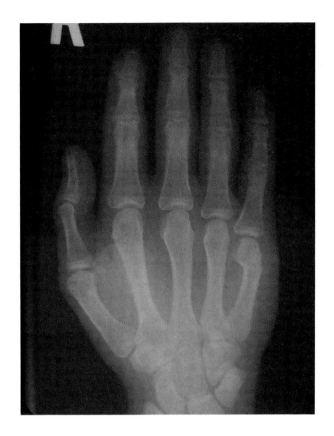

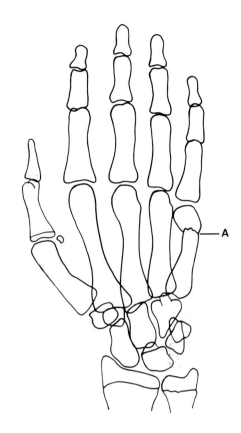

77   **Trans-scapho perilunar dislocation of the**
◄   **carpus.**

   (a)   *PA view.*
       On the PA view, the lunate (A) looks
       triangular. The clues that this is not lunate
       dislocation are the presence of an associated
       scaphoid fracture (B) and widening of the
       ulnar aspect of the wrist joint (C).

   (b)   *Lateral view.*
       The lateral view shows that the lunate (A) is
       in normal alignment with the radius (D). The
       rest of the carpus (E) is displaced posteriorly.

78   **Fracture of the 5th metacarpal.**
      This is a common injury (A), often sustained
      in throwing a punch.

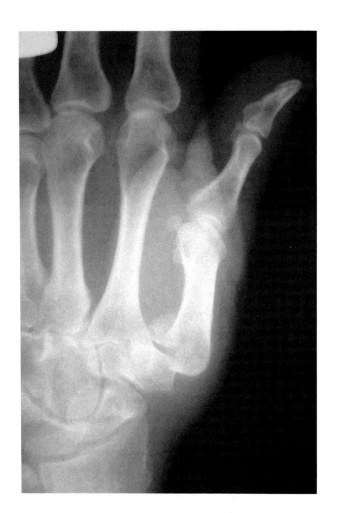

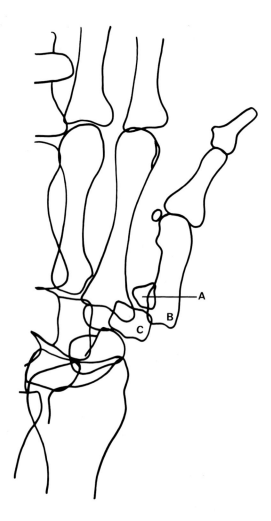

79 **Fracture/dislocation of the 1st metacarpal.**
This injury is known as Bennett's
fracture/dislocation. There is a fracture of the
base of the 1st metacarpal with separation of
the medial fragment (A). The base of the 1st
metacarpal (B) is dislocated with respect to
the trapezium (C).

3: MISCELLANEOUS CONDITIONS INCLUDING AVASCULAR NECROSIS AND OSTEOCHONDRITIS

Many of the conditions illustrated in this section were considered formerly to be of uncertain aetiology. It is likely that most of them are post-traumatic, particularly those loosely labelled as 'osteochondritis'.

Avascular necrosis also plays a part in many of them and is itself often post-traumatic, particularly in the femoral head and scaphoid.

Other conditions illustrated, for instance, Paget's disease, remain of unknown aetiology.

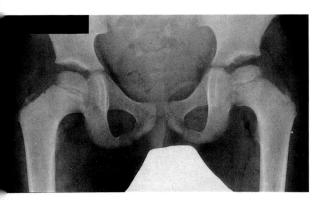

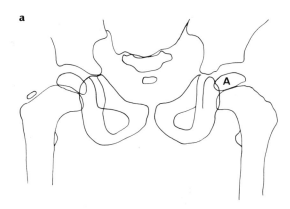

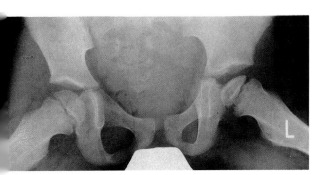

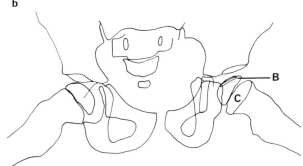

80   Perthe's disease.
This condition of uncertain aetiology affects mainly males between the ages of 2 and 14 years with a peak incidence between 4 and 5 years. It may be a form of avascular necrosis. It is bilateral in about 10 per cent of cases. Bone maturation is retarded. In early cases, a subarticular lucent fissure is seen in the femoral head.

(a)   *AP view.*
In this example, the left femoral head (A) is small, indicating retarded maturation.

(b)   *'Frog'—lateral view.*
The small size of the left femoral head is more clearly seen.
A subarticular lucent fissure (B) is present and there is also a lucent metaphyseal band (C), a common accompaniment.

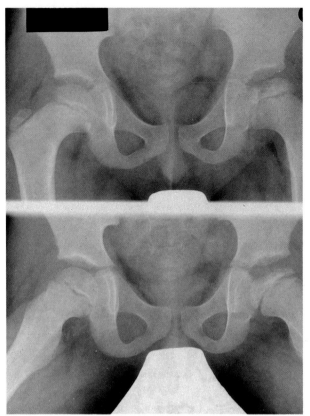

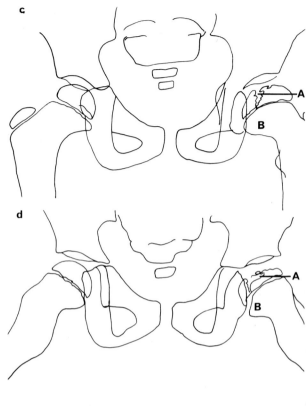

(c & d) Same patient—15 months later.
    The flattening of the femoral head has
    increased and the fissuring has progressed

to fragmentation (A). There is secondary
widening of the metaphysis (B).

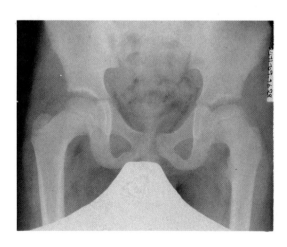

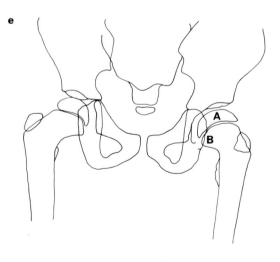

(e)   *Sixteen months later.*
    Healing has occurred. There is still residual
    flattening of the femoral head (A) and the
    metaphysis (B) remains widened. Different

factors influence the completeness of
healing but, in general, the earlier the onset
of the disease, the better the prognosis.

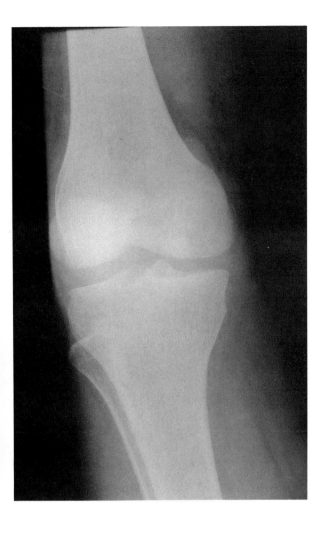

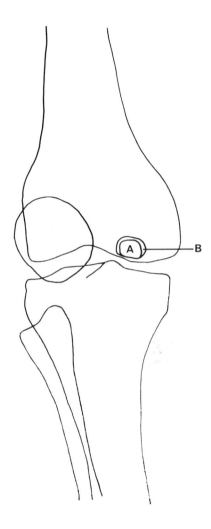

81   **Osteochondritis dissecans.**
There is separation of a fragment of bone
and cartilage from the surface of a convex
joint, usually the condyle of the femur. The
fragment may become an intra-articular
loose body. The condition is probably of
traumatic aetiology.

(a)   AP view.
In this example, in the knee, a fragment of
bone (A) is separated from the medial
femoral condyle and has a well-defined
lucent margin (B).

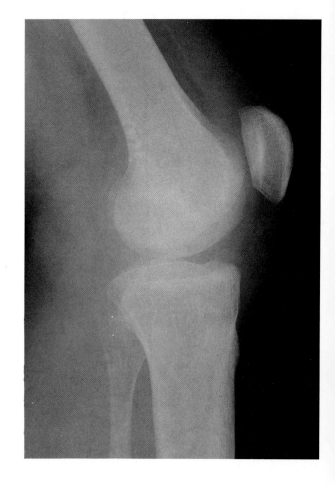

(b) *Lateral view.*
The fragment (A) and its margin (B) are
seen more clearly. This is one of the many
examples of the need to take views of a joint
at right angles to each other.

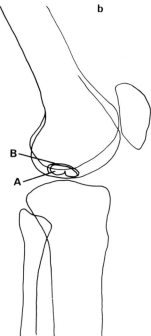

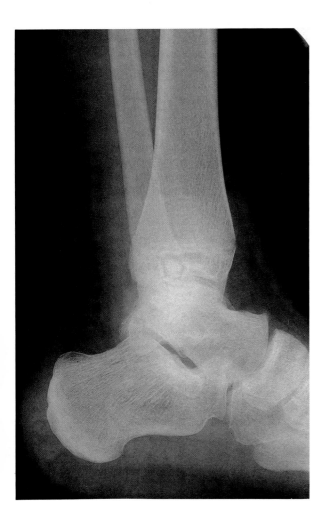

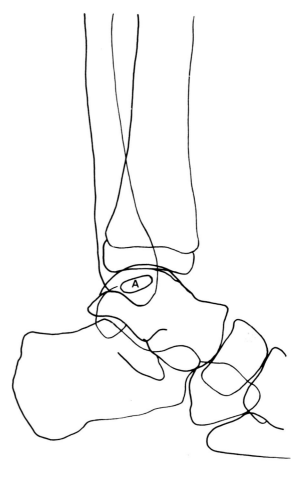

82   **Osteochondritis dissecans of the talus.**

(a)   *Lateral view.*
This view shows a fragment of bone (A) separated from the superior surface of the talus.

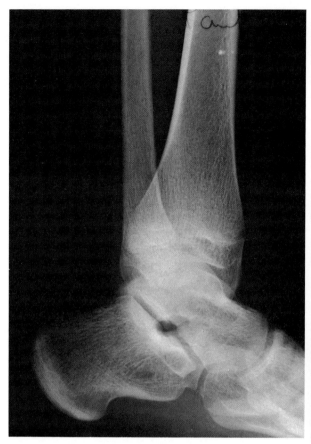

(b) *Oblique view.*
An oblique view shows the fragment (A)
and its lucent margin (B) more clearly.

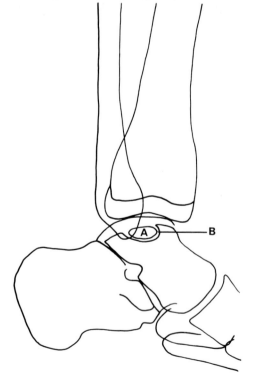

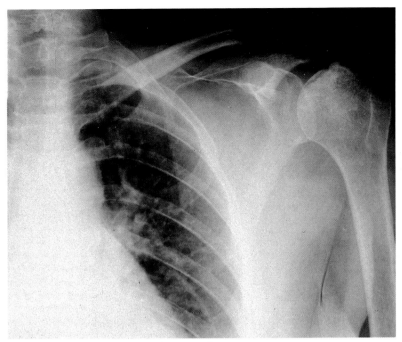

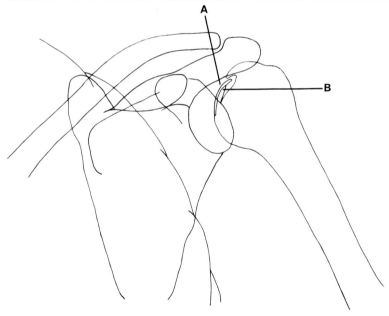

83 Avascular necrosis of the left shoulder.
There is a dense fragment of the humeral articular surface (A) separated from the rest of the humeral head by a narrow lucent line (B). This type of lesion occurs in dysbaric osteonecrosis (Caisson disease).

111

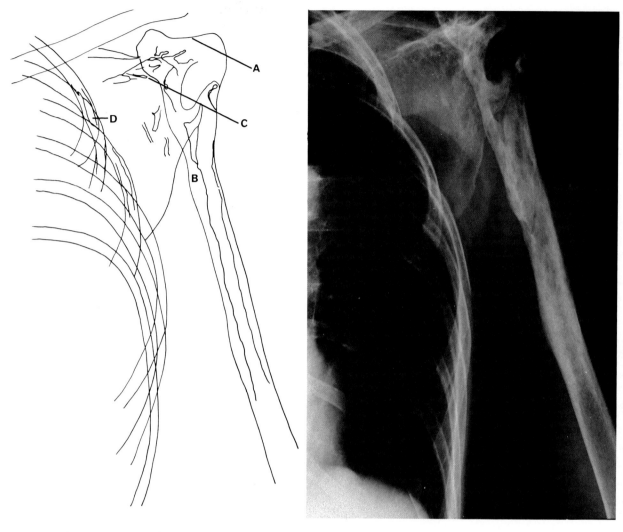

84 **Radiation osteonecrosis.**
The radiological changes are a consequence
of bone death, demineralization and (in the
immature skeleton) retarded bone growth.
In this example, there is radiation necrosis
of the left upper humerus, scapula and ribs
following radiotherapy for breast cancer.

The humeral head (A) is deficient. There is
disordered architecture with dense,
irregular bony sclerosis in the humerus (B),
scapula (C) and ribs (D).
These appearances should not be mistaken
for metastases, which are generally more
destructive.

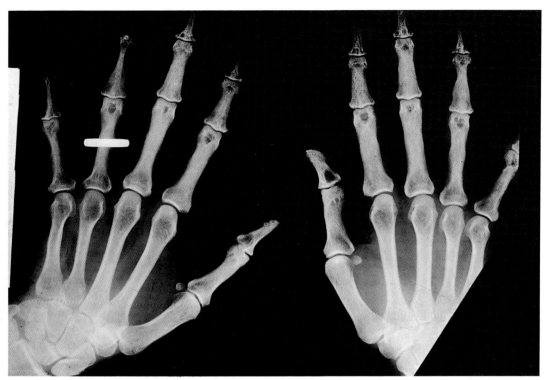

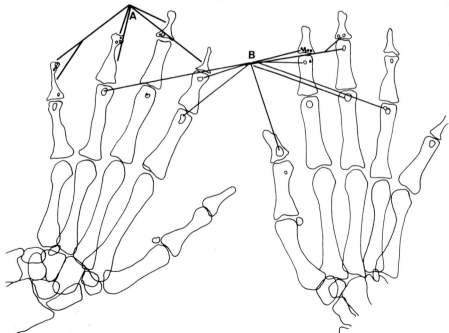

85   Sarcoidosis of bone.
Sarcoidosis is a non-caseating granulomatous disease. Its chest manifestations are better known than its skeletal ones but bone changes occur in about 10 per cent of cases.
The lesions are generally well-defined and lytic and involve the metacarpals and phalanges. Other alterations in bone texture may occur.
This example, in the hand, shows erosion of the terminal phalanges (A) and lucent lesions at the ends of the phalanges (B).

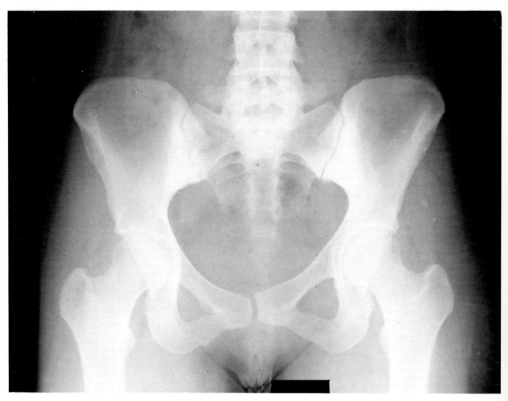

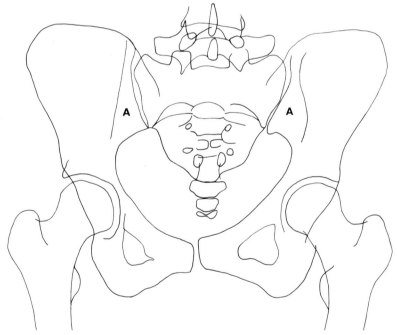

86   Osteitis condensans ilii.
There is sclerosis (A) of the iliac aspects of the sacro-iliac joints. The joints themselves are normal. The condition is usually bilateral and occurs in young women. It is probably secondary to stress during parturition. Unilateral lesions may occur in patients with an abnormal contralateral hip.

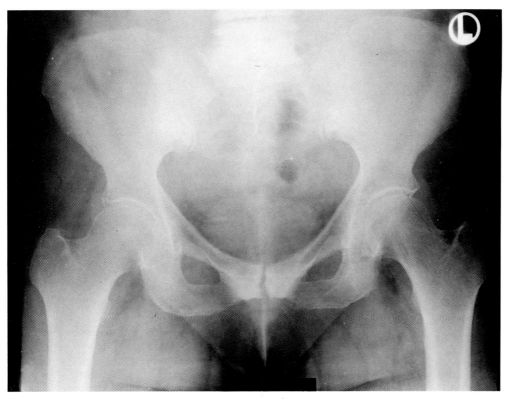

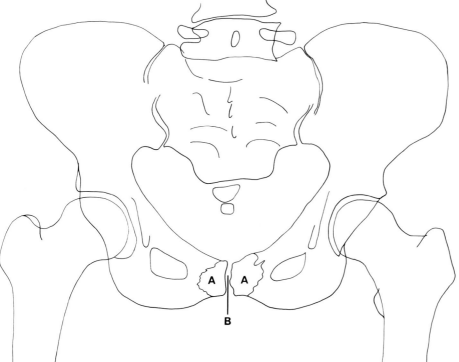

87 **Osteitis pubis.**
There is sclerosis (A) of both sides of the pubic symphysis (B). This is another example of a stress lesion and it may occur in athletes as well as after parturition.

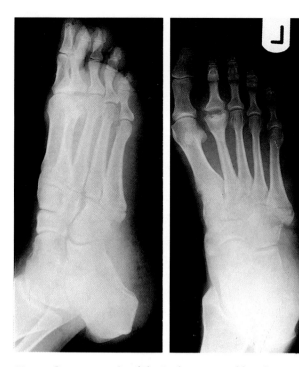
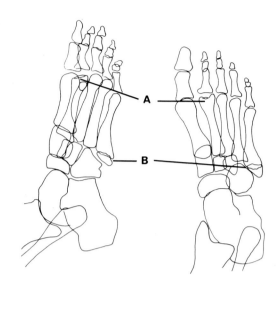

88 Osteonecrosis of the 2nd metatarsal head (Freiberg's disease).
This and other forms of 'osteochondritis' of epiphyses and small bones are probably post-traumatic. The second metatarsal head is flattened and sclerotic (A). The patient also has a fracture of the base of the fifth metatarsal (B).

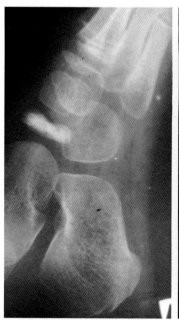
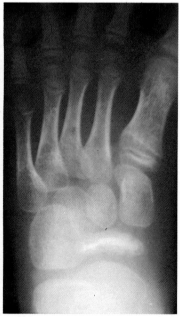
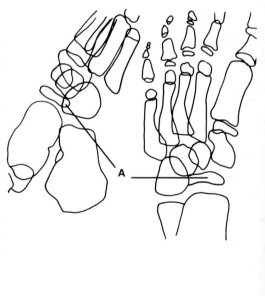

89 Osteochondritis of the navicular (Kohler's disease).
The navicular is small, flattened and dense (A).

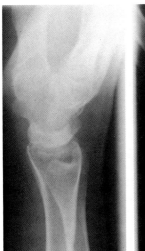
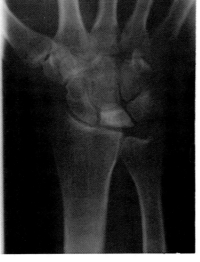

90   Osteochondritis of the lunate (Keinbock's disease).

This is probably also post traumatic. The lunate (Λ) is small and sclerotic.

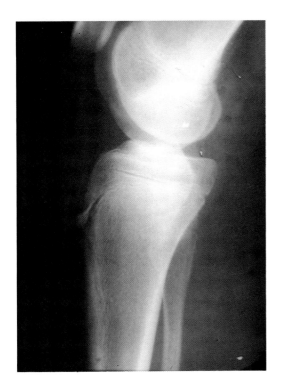
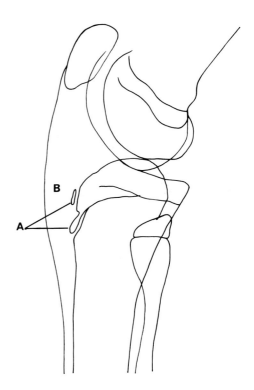

91   Osteochondritis of the tibial apophysis (Osgood-Schlatter's disease).
This is probably an example of a chronic avulsion injury related to the attachment of the patellar ligament into the tibial

tuberosity (A). There is a dense, fragmented upper tibial apophysis (A). There is associated soft tissue swelling (B) and tenderness, best assessed clinically.

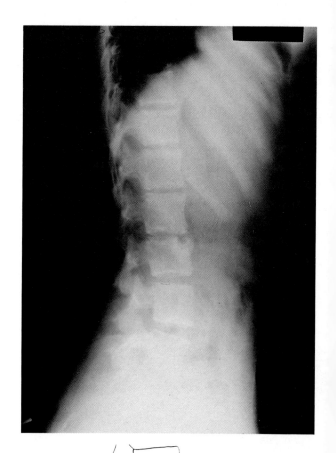

92   Localised osteochondritis of the spine.
There is a lucent defect (A) with a sclerotic
border (B) in the upper, anterior border of
LV3. Such lesions are of uncertain aetiology
and should not be confused with infective
lesions. They may have a post-traumatic
aetiology or be related to Scheuermann's
disease.

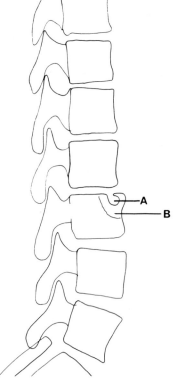

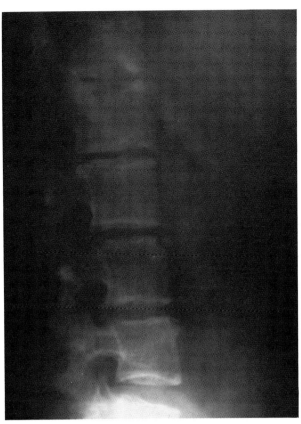

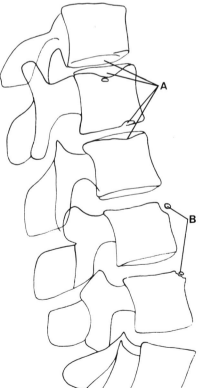

93   **Scheuermann's disease.**
The hallmark of this condition, which
affects the spines of adolescents, is
Schmorrl's node (A). It is thought to be due
to herniation of the nucleus purposus into
the adjacent vertebral body. The other
changes, such as irregularity of the
antero-superior parts of the vertebral
bodies (B) and eventual kyphosis are
thought to be secondary.

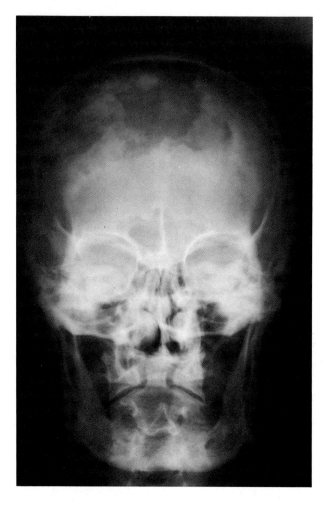

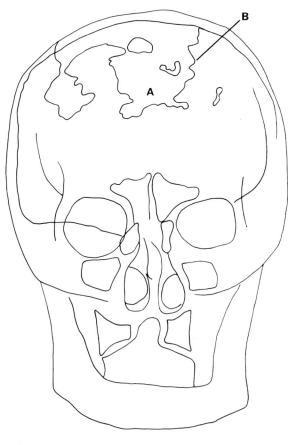

94   **Paget's disease.**
This is a relatively common bone disorder
of unknown aetiology affecting the
middle-aged and old. It is often a chance
radiographic finding.
There are three main radiological
appearances which may co-exist in the
same patient, or even in the same bone.
They are:

      1   The active, or lytic stage
      2   The spongy stage
      3   The amorphous stage

Examples of all three stages are shown in
the following illustrations.

(a)   Lytic stage.
     Osteoporosis circumscripta of the skull.
     There is a large, lytic frontal lesion (A) with
     irregular margins (B).

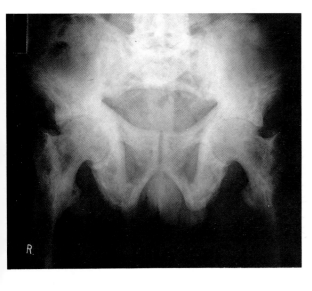
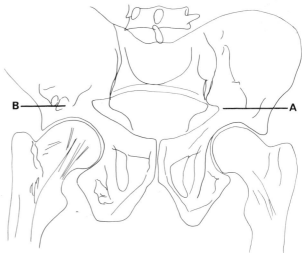

95 **Paget's disease of the pelvis.**

(a) *AP view.*
There is marked bone expansion. The pelvic brim (A) is flattened, secondary to the bone softening which occurs in Paget's disease. Both the spongy (B) and amorphous changes are present.

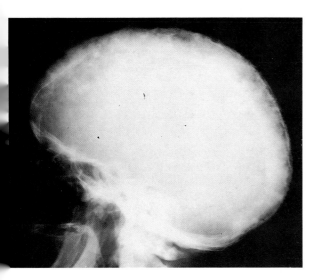
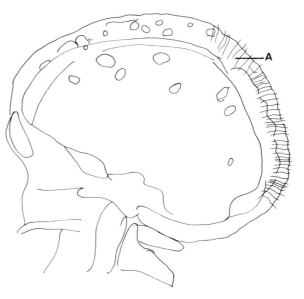

(b) *Skull of the same patient.*
The skull vault is grossly thickened and it is mainly the amorphous stage of the disease which is present although some spongy changes (A) are seen, mainly in the posterior parietal region.

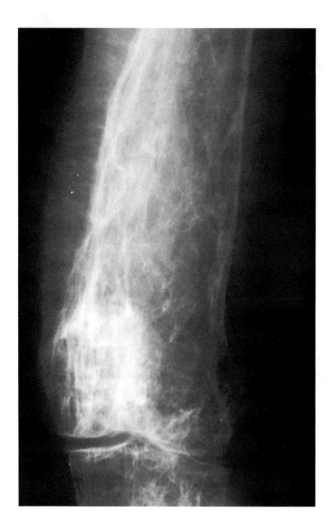

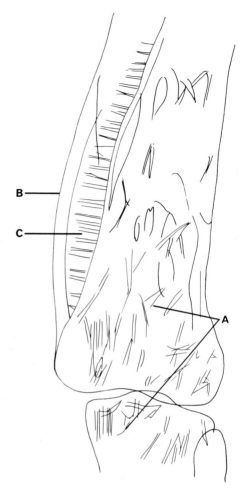

96   Paget's disease of femur with sarcomatous change.
The femur and proximal tibia show the typical expansion and coarse pattern of the spongy stage of Paget's disease (A). In addition, there is soft tissue swelling (B) over the distal aspect of the distal femur with periosteal new bone formation seen as 'sun-ray spiculation', perpendicular to the cortex (C). Such an appearance indicates sarcomatous change.

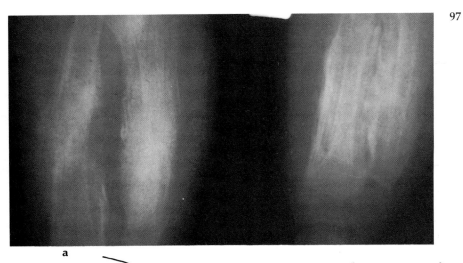

a

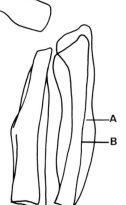
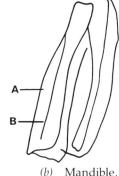

97 **Infantile cortical hyperostosis (Caffey's disease).** This is a condition of unknown aetiology. The three cardinal features are hyper-irritability, soft tissue swelling and cortical bony thickening. The swellings usually resolve within weeks or months. Occasionally, the condition becomes chronic and leads to deformity.

(a) Left radius of ulna showing gross periosteal thickening along the bone shafts (A) outside the original cortex (B).

(b) Mandible, again showing gross periosteal thickening (A) outside the cortex.

b

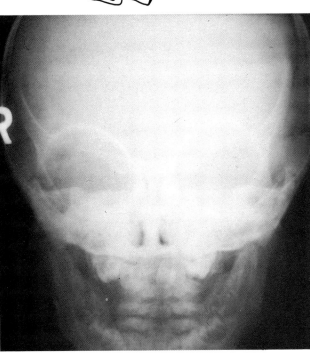
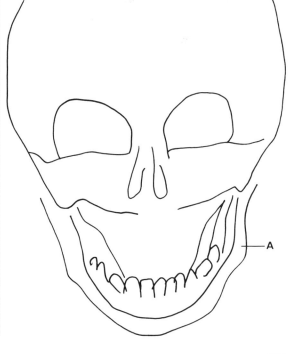

4: INFECTIONS OF BONE

The radiological changes in bone infections are those of hyperaemia, bone destruction and attempts at repair. The full radiological picture of osteomyelitis is seldom seen in developed countries thanks to prompt antibiotic treatment. The classical appearances of established osteomyelitis are:

1   Sequestrum formation. This is denser, dead bone within the shaft.
2   A cloaca, which is a drainage hole in the cortex through which pus escapes. It is sometimes surgically induced.
3   Involucrum, which is periosteal new bone surrounding the shaft.

It is important to treat suspected osteomyelitis on clinical grounds as it takes at least 10 to 14 days for radiological changes to occur.

Damaged bone is more prone to infection, for instance, after open trauma or in the bone infarcts of sickle cell disease. The infecting organism cannot be determined from the radiograph except in some specific cases such as tuberculosis, when the findings may be characteristic.

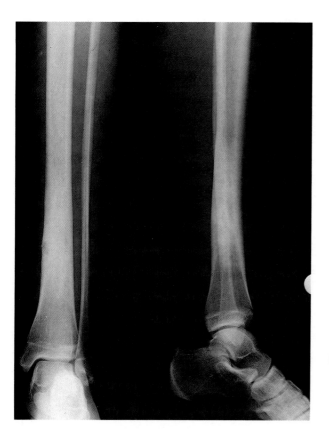
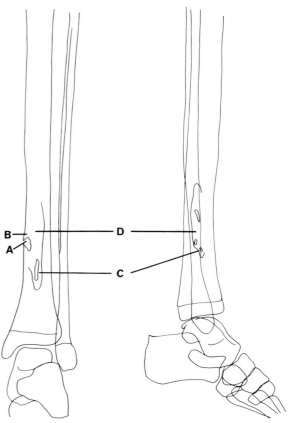

98   **Osteomyelitis of tibia.**

(a)   *AP and lateral views.*
There is a small, peripheral, lucent defect (A) breaching the cortex (B). An ill-defined lucency is seen within the medulla (C). The surrounding bone is slightly sclerotic (D).

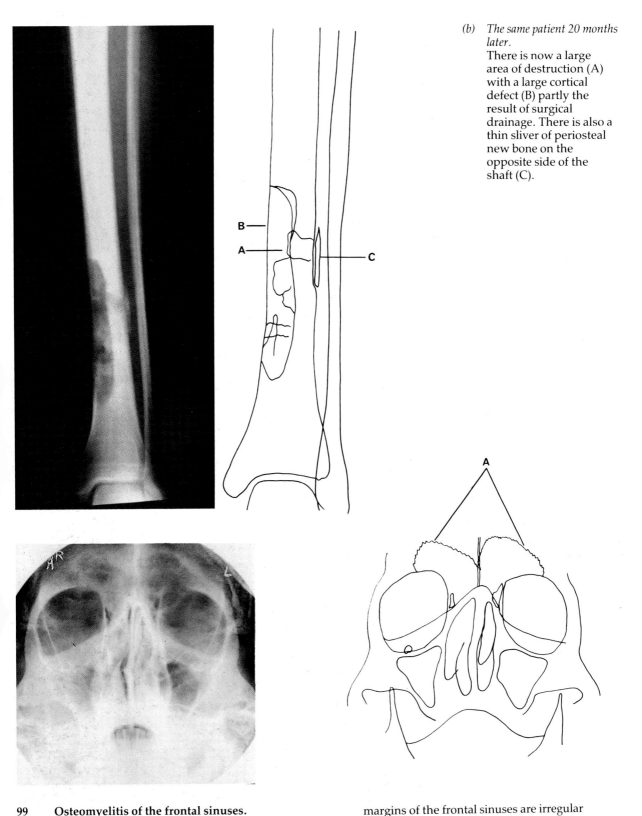

(b) *The same patient 20 months later.*
There is now a large area of destruction (A) with a large cortical defect (B) partly the result of surgical drainage. There is also a thin sliver of periosteal new bone on the opposite side of the shaft (C).

99   Osteomyelitis of the frontal sinuses.
This is a complication of sinusitis. The margins of the frontal sinuses are irregular with some sclerosis (A).

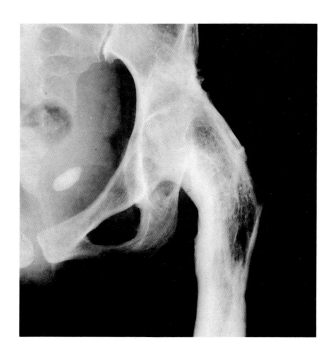
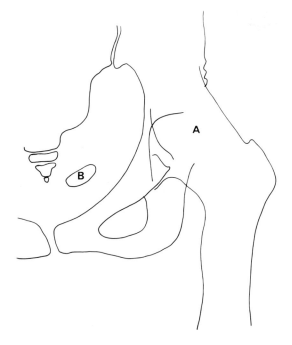

100   Old osteomyelitis and septic arthritis of the hip.
Both the joint and the surrounding bones have been chronically infected. The end result is complete bony ankylosis of the hip (A). There is also a bladder calculus (B).

101   Brodie's abscess of the distal tibia. ▶
This is chronic, low grade infection manifested as a central, well-defined lucent defect (A) with a sclerotic margin (B). There is slight periosteal reaction (C).

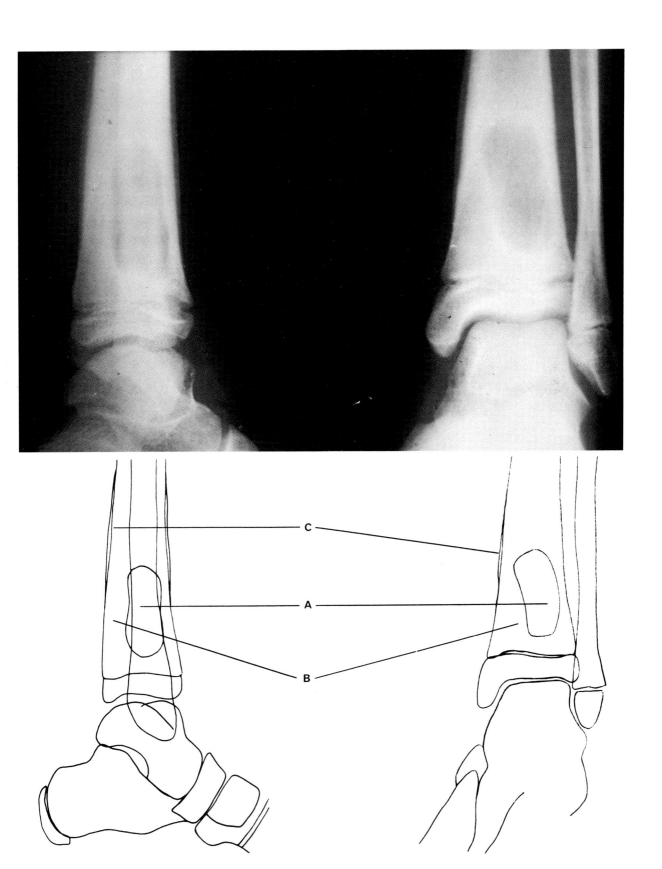

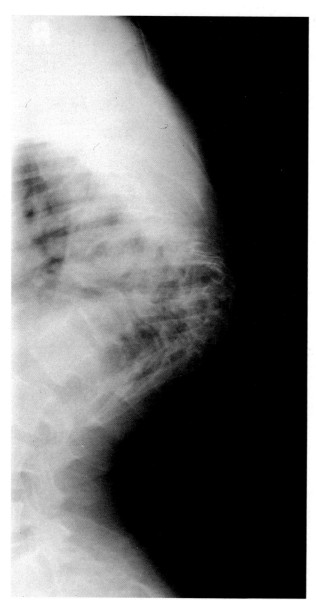

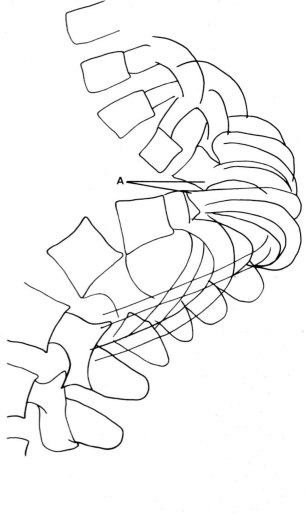

102   Tuberculosis.
Tuberculosis has a slower progression than osteomyelitis and there is usually radiological evidence of disease at first presentation. The presence of calcification is very strong evidence of tuberculosis.

(a)   Spinal tuberculosis, lateral view.
Spinal tuberculosis tends to involve the disc margins first, though it may start in a vertebral body. This lateral view of the thoracic spine shows collapse with anterior wedging of DV10, 11 and 12 (A) and consequent severe kyphosis.

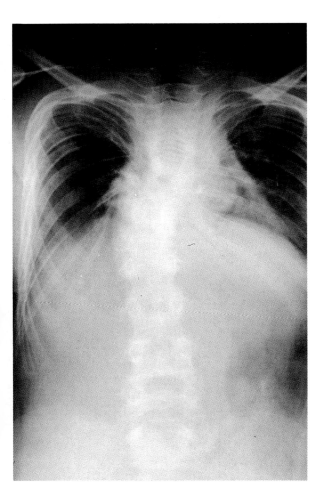

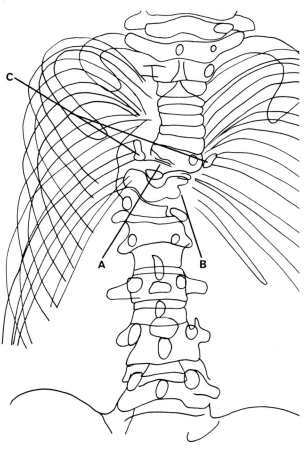

(b) *AP view.*
The abnormal lower thoracic vertebral
bodies (A) cannot be seen clearly. There is
scoliosis (B) and the posterior ends of the
ribs are crowded due to kyphosis.
Calcification is seen in paravertebral cold
abscess (C).

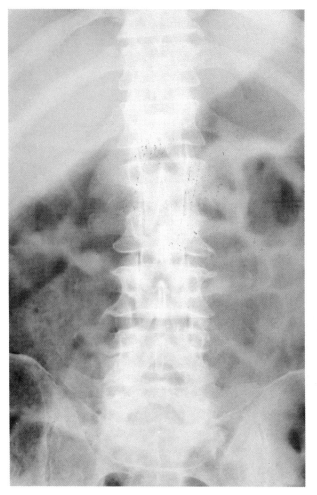

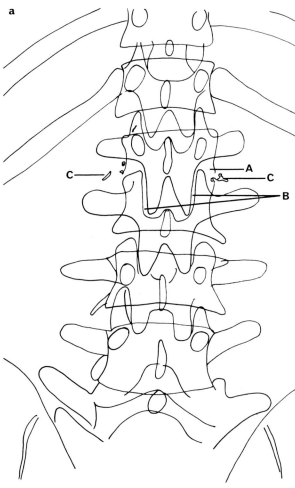

103   Tuberculosis of lumbar spine.

(a) *AP view.*
The margins of LV1 and 2 (A) are indistinct and the apophyseal joints (B) can be seen more clearly through the partly destroyed bodies than at other levels. There is faint paravertebral soft tissue calcification (C).

(b) *Coned lateral view.*
There is fusion of LV1 and 2 with virtual obliteration of the disc space (A). LV1 and 2 are reduced in height compared with the adjacent vertebrae, due to destruction and collapse along their adjacent margins.

(c) *Cervical spine of the same patient.*
There are tiny erosions of the antero-superior (A) and antero-inferior margins of CV4 and of the antero-superior margin of CV5 (B). Taken on their own, these appearances cannot be distinguished from pyogenic infection. However, the site and lack of sclerosis are suggestive of tuberculosis.
The lumbar spine lesion with its associated calcification is confirmatory.
Multifocal spinal tuberculosis is rare in Britain but may be seen in developing countries, particularly in debilitated children.

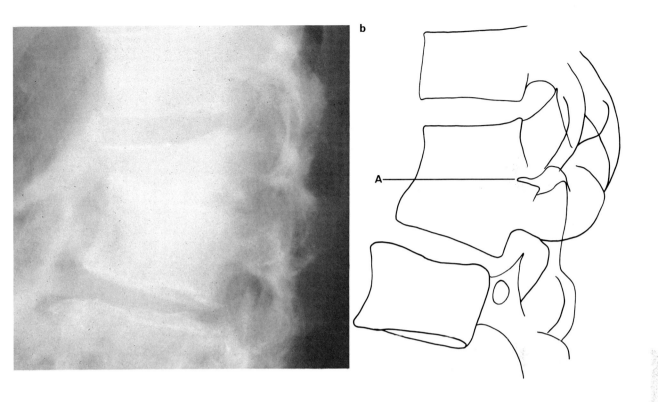

b

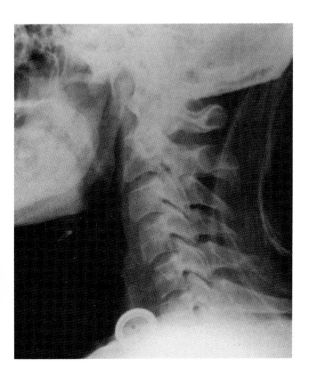

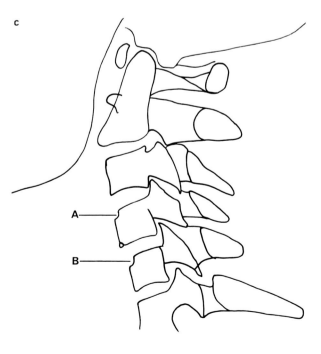

c

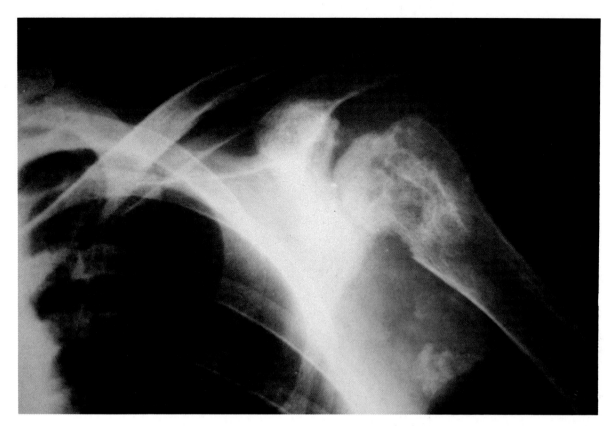

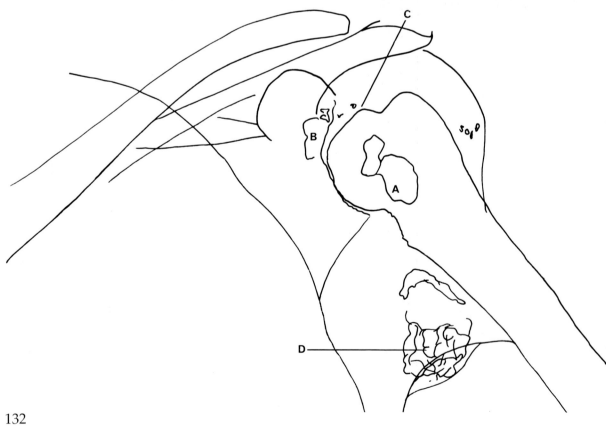

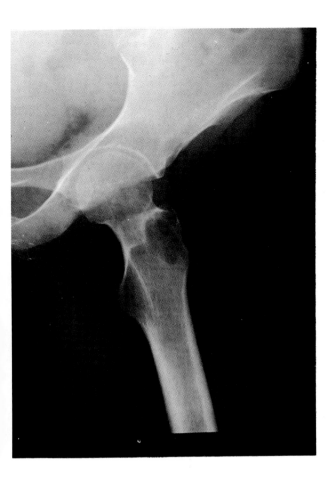
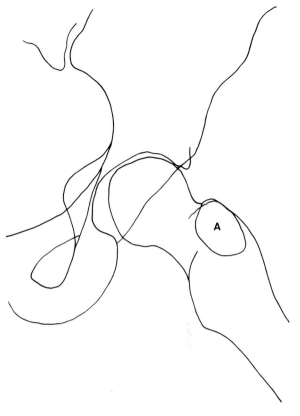

105   Tuberculosis of the left greater trochanter.
There is a well-defined, cystic defect (A) in the greater trochanter. The greater trochanter is a recognised site of this fairly indolent form of the disease.

104   Tuberculosis of right shoulder.
◀   There are erosions round the anatomical neck of the humerus (A) and in the glenoid (B). This metaphyseal involvement is relatively common in joint tuberculosis and the proximal humeral articular surface (C) is reasonably well-preserved. It is also relatively common for both sides of the joint to be involved. The presence of calcification (D) in the large soft tissue swelling is characteristic.

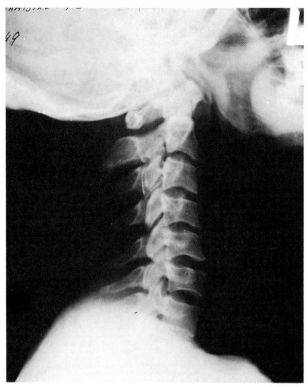
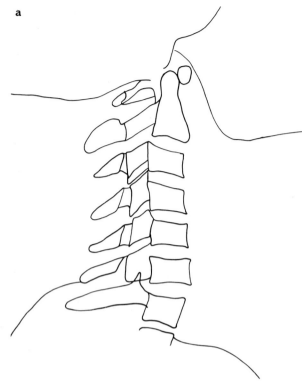

106 Brucellosis.

The bony appearances of brucellosis are not specific but the diagnosis should be considered, particularly in a bony infection of the spine, in groups at risk such as veterinary surgeons and dairy farm workers.

The following examples show progression of the disease in the cervical spine.

(a) *Normal cervical spine.*

(b) *Two months later.*
There is marked destruction along the C4/5 disc margins (A).

(c) *Eighteen months later.*
There is complete ankylosis of C4 and 5 (B).

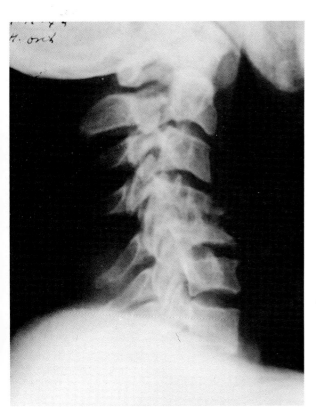

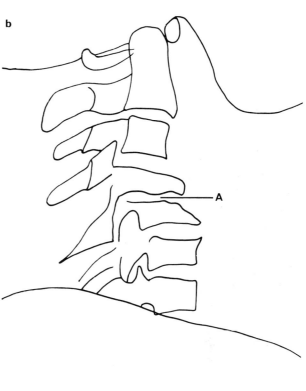

b

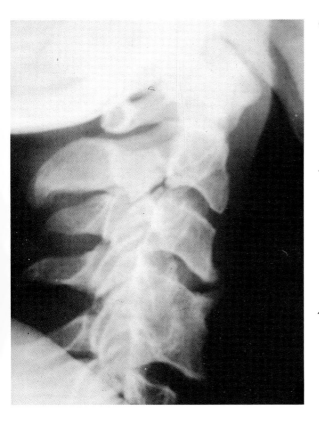

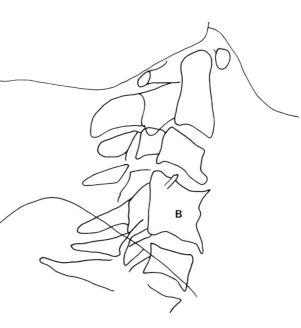

c

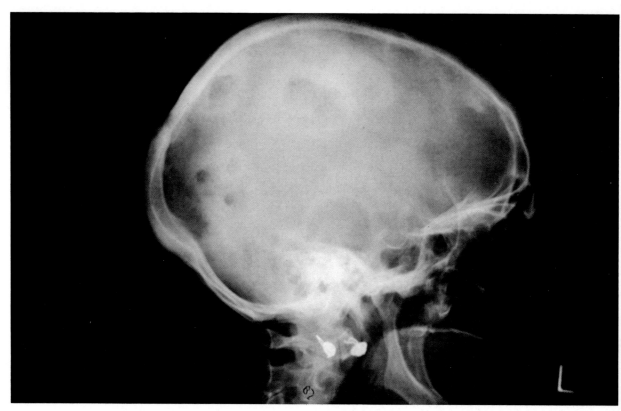

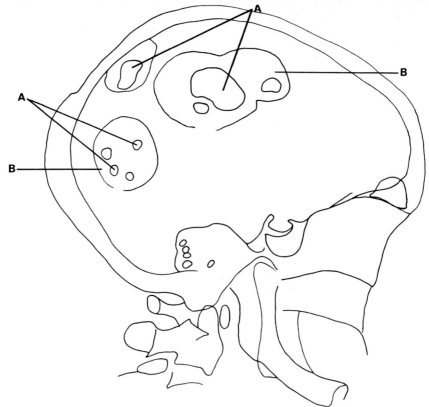

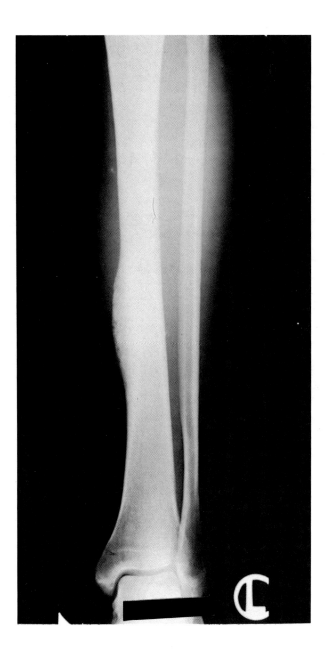

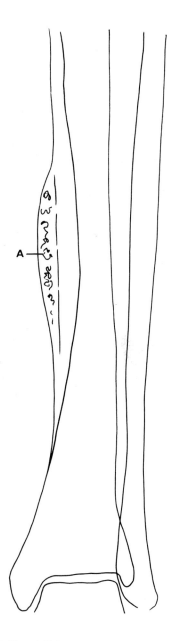

107   Syphilis.
◄
If bony abnormality occurs in acquired
syphilis, it is usually in the tertiary stage of
the disease. Radiologically, there tends to
be a combination of osteolysis and new
bone formation which may mimic a
neoplasm. Bone syphilis is exceptionally
rare nowadays. The first example shows
syphilis of the skull. There are multiple
lucent lesions (A) with thick sclerotic
margins.

108   Syphilis of tibia.
There is dense periosteal new bone
formation with irregular patchy
radiolucencies within it (A).

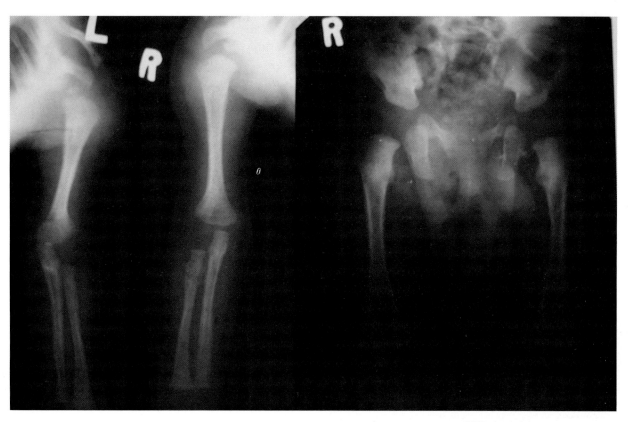

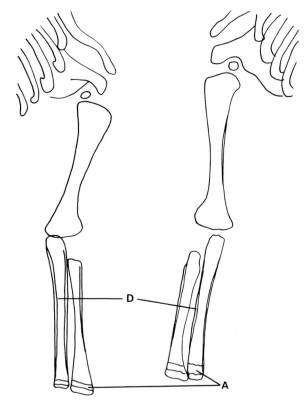

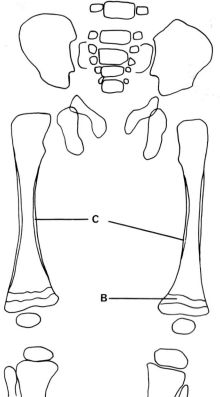

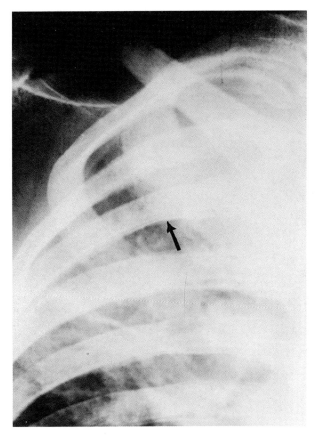
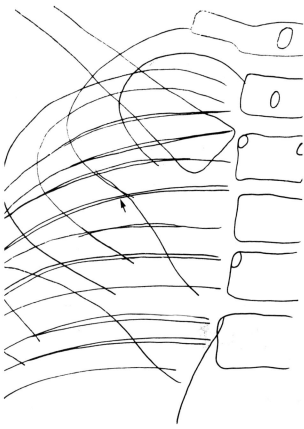

110   Actinomycosis.
This rather rare fungus infection tends to affect the mandible or abdomen. Lesions in the pleura and ribs are probably secondary to mandibular foci. Actinomycosis is mainly destructive in bone. On the PA film of this patient, the appearances looked just like

right upper lobe pneumonia. However, on the coned upper rib view, there is periosteal reaction along the posterior aspects of the 3rd, 4th (arrowed), 5th, 6th and 7th ribs. Such an appearance would rarely, if ever, occur in bacterial pneumonia.

109   Congenital syphilis.
◄   This is not as rare as acquired syphilitic bone disease and is seen relatively frequently in neonates in developing countries. It is usual to find the metaphyses of the long bones affected.

This example shows typical changes in the upper and lower limbs. Lucent metaphyseal bands are best seen at the wrists (A) and knees (B). Periosteal reaction is present and is most clearly seen along the femoral (C) and ulnar shafts (D).

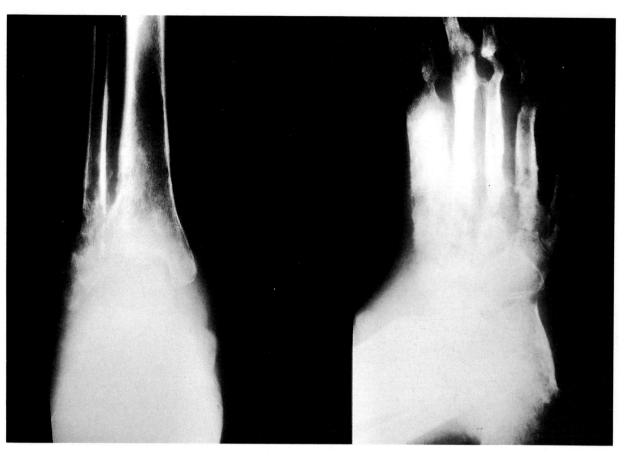

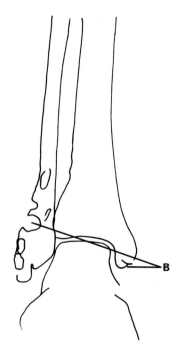

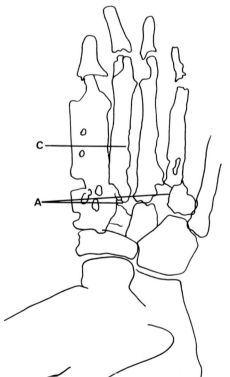

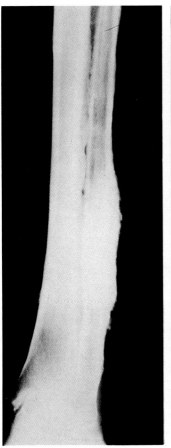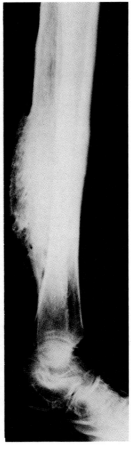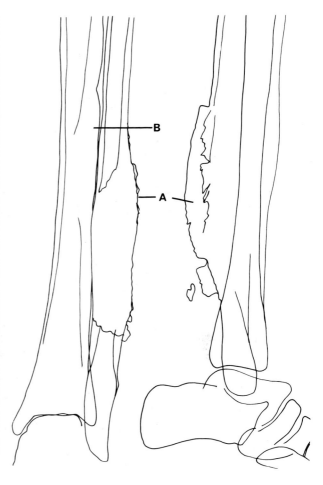

112 **Tropical ulcer.**
The bone changes are secondary to ulceration, often of many years standing, in the skin and soft tissues. It occurs in the lower limb.
Periosteal reaction occurs first and builds up over months and years into periosteal and cortical thickening.
In this example, there is florid cortical bony thickening (A), mainly on the postero-lateral aspect of the fibula. There is also tibial cortical thickening (B), particularly along its fibular border.

111 **Mycetoma ('Madura foot').**
◄ This fungal infection, rare in countries where shoes are worn, may be caused by several different fungi of the maduromycetes, actinomycetes and streptomycetes group. It usually affects the foot and occasionally other parts of the lower limb.
In the advanced stage, practically nothing else gives such a florid, destructive appearance. There is gross, irregular destruction of the bones of the foot (A) and ankle (B) with some irregular, sclerotic, periosteal reaction (C).

5: DISEASES OF JOINTS

The radiological manifestations of joint disease are seen in the joint spaces, adjacent bone surfaces and surrounding soft tissues.

Arthritis may be destructive, as in rheumatoid or septic arthritis, or productive with new bone formation in osteoarthritis. Osteoarthrosis is probably a better term than osteoarthritis as the appearances are the result of mechanical joint wear rather than inflammation.

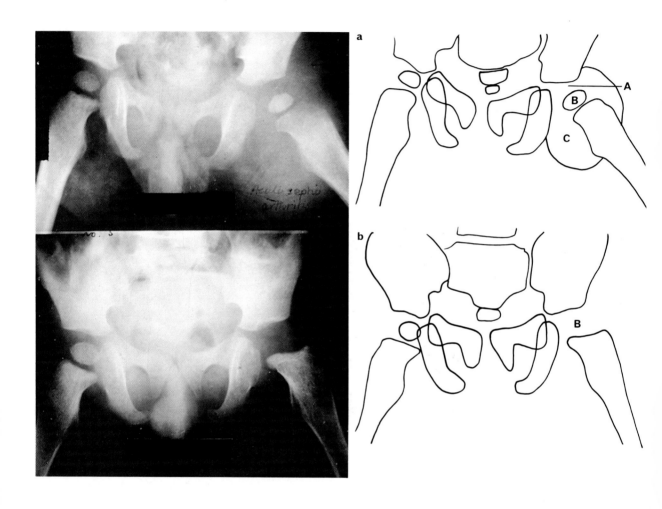

113   **Acute septic arthritis.**
The full-blown picture of septic arthritis is now comparatively rare as antibiotic treatment is usually started in the early stages. Often, all that is seen is an effusion into the joint, with widening of the joint space and distension of the capsule. The later stages of bony destruction, joint space narrowing and eventual ankylosis are now rare.
This example of septic arthritis of the hips is taken from the early days of antibiotic therapy.

(a)   *Early.*
On the first film, there is a little widening of the hip joint space (A) with displacement of the femoral head (B) laterally. The femur is held in abduction. There is a large joint effusion which is seen as a surrounding soft tissue shadow (C).

(b)   *Late.*
A film taken six months later shows complete destruction of the femoral head (B).

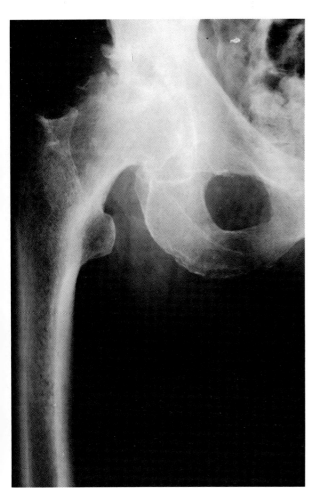
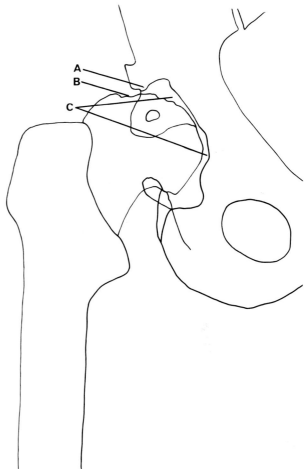

114 **Septic arthritis in an adult hip.**
This is a lower grade lesion with some irregular, marginal sclerosis (A). There is irregular destruction of the lateral aspect of the femoral head (B) and marked destruction of the acetabulum (C).

115   Rheumatoid arthritis.
In this common and well-known erosive
polyarthritis, clinical symptoms may
precede abnormal radiological findings by
several weeks or months. The place of
radiology in the initial diagnosis is,
therefore, limited and clinical appearances
and serological changes are more
important. However, radiological findings
may be seen at first presentation and
should be recognised.
The metatarso-phalangeal and
metacarpo-phalangeal joints are usually
involved first but no synovial joint is
exempt. The first example shows typical
changes in a hand.
A   There are marked erosions of the
     second, third and fourth metacarpal
     heads with considerable bony
     destruction.
B   The proximal interphalangeal joints are
     narrowed with deformity of the fifth
     (C).
D   Small carpal erosions are seen on the
     scaphoid and capitate.
E   There is some juxta-articular
     osteoporosis.

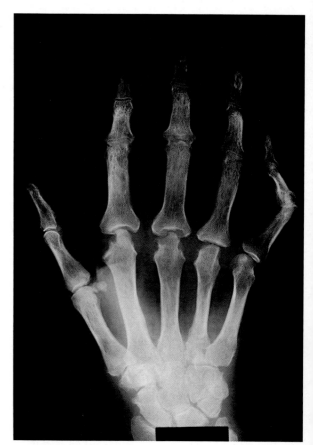

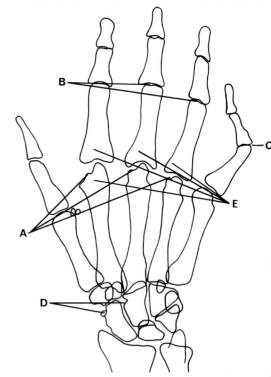

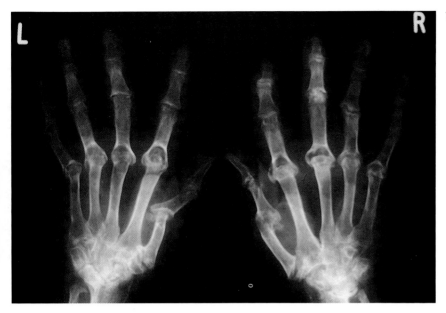

Rheumatoid arthritis mutilans of the hands.
Not all patients progress to this severe, destructive stage of the disease. All of the joints of the wrist, carpus and hands are involved.

A   The wrist joints are narrow with irregular margins.

B   Both ulnar styloids are eroded away and there is a narrow, tapered distal right ulna.

C   The carpal joints are grossly narrowed with irregular margins.

D   The metacarpo-phalangeal joints are grossly eroded. The right first metacarpo-phalangeal joint is fused (E).

F   The proximal and terminal metacarpo-phalangeal joints are also affected.

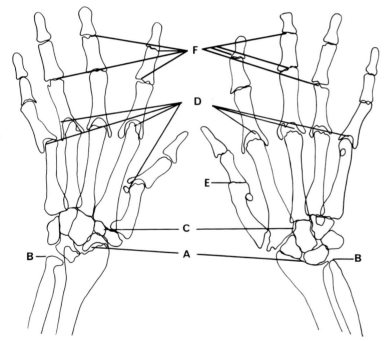

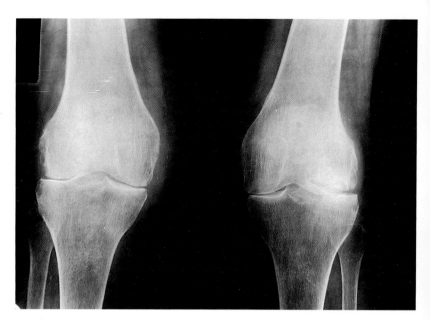

117 Rheumatoid arthritis of knees.
Soft tissue swelling due to synovial thickening (A) is usually apparent clinically and radiologically when the knee is affected by rheumatoid arthritis. There is also bilateral joint space narrowing (B) and erosion of the left lateral femoral condyle (C).

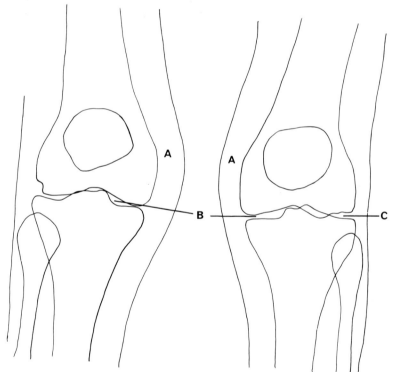

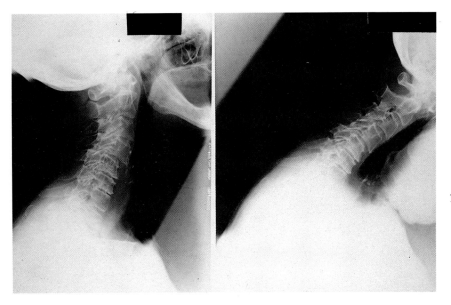

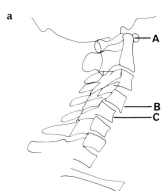

a

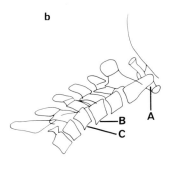

b

118 Rheumatoid arthritis of the cervical spine.
The atlanto-axial joint is an important site of rheumatoid arthritis as dislocation can lead to neurological symptoms or even death.

(a) *Cervical spine in extension.*

(b) *Cervical spine in flexion.*
The gap (A) between the anterior arch of the atlas and the odontoid peg is much wider on the flexion view (B), indicating joint instability. There is also subluxation of CV4 (B) on CV5 (C). This has not increased in flexion and is probably stable.

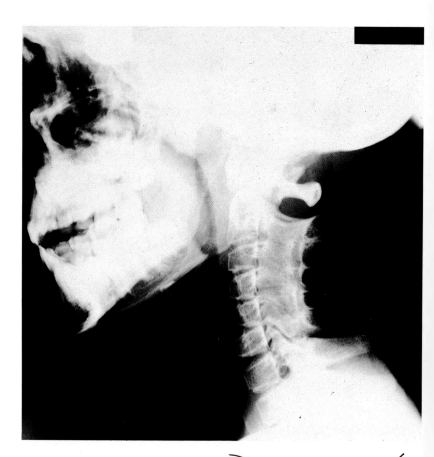

119 **Juvenile rheumatoid arthritis—Still's disease.** There are usually more systemic abnormalities than in adult rheumatoid arthritis. These include fever, splenomegaly, lymphadenopathy and pericarditis. Unlike the adult form, large joints may be involved first. Although many cases resolve without serious sequelae, the fact that growing bone ends are involved may mean eventual deformity. In the spine, ankylosis may be the end result. This example shows small vertebral bodies (A) with fused neural arches (B). Fusion of both bodies and arches may simulate a congenital spinal fusion.

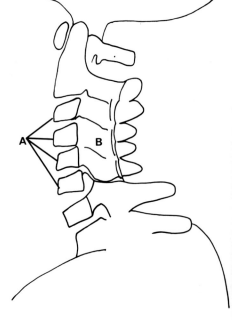

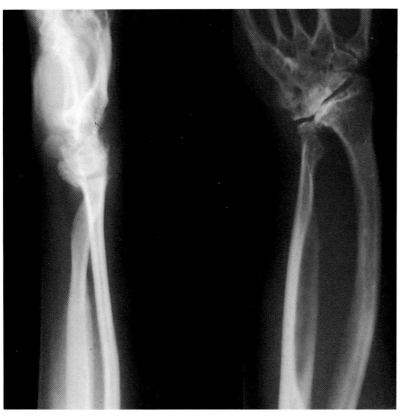

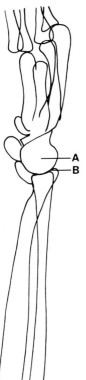 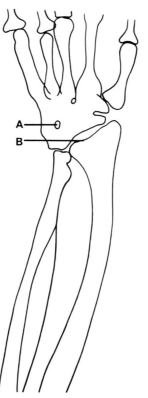

120   Juvenile rheumatoid arthritis.
Right wrist and hand. In this late stage of the disease, there is marked deformity with fusion of the carpals (A). The wrist joint is deformed and has irregular margins (B).

149

121   Osteoarthritis.
This is a degenerative and not an inflammatory process. As opposed to the various forms of inflammatory arthritis, it is productive of new bone rather than destructive, although joint space narrowing is a feature due to cartilage loss. New bone formation is seen as sclerosis and osteophyte formation along joint margins, particularly of large, weight-bearing joints. An erosive form does occur in the hands but it is accompanied by osteophytes (Heberden's nodes) and affects the terminal interphalangeal joints which are generally spared by rheumatoid arthritis.

Osteoarthritis is usually idiopathic but is often secondary to trauma or pre-existing joint disease. When it is superimposed on old rheumatoid arthritis, there may be some diagnostic difficulty but the presence of osteophytes suggests secondary osteoarthritis.

The first example shows typical osteoarthritis of the hips. The joint spaces (A) are narrowed. The margins are sclerotic (B) and there is osteophyte formation (C). Osteophytes are also present at the disc margins (D), indicating degenerative change, or spondylosis, of the lumbar spine.

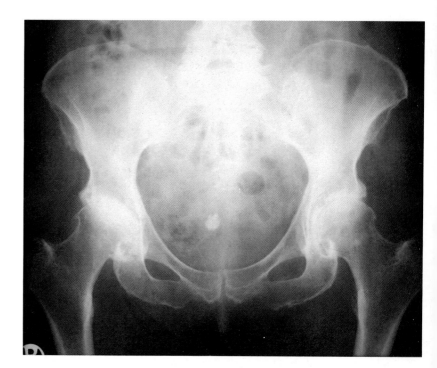

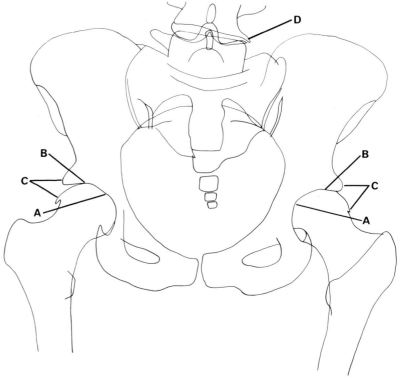

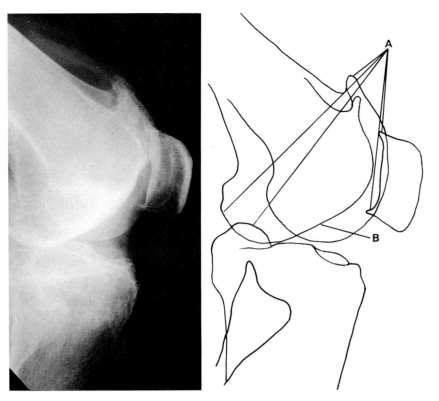

122   Osteoarthritis of the left knee.

(a) *Lateral view.*
Prominent osteophyte formation (A) is shown on the margins of the patello-femoral joint and posterior aspect of the knee joint. The medial femoral condyle is sclerotic and slightly flattened (B).

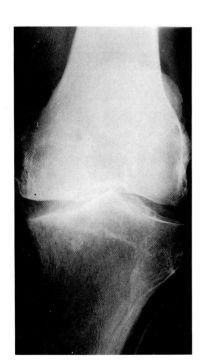
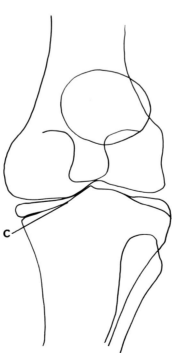

(b) *AP view.*
The central part of the joint space is narrowed with sclerotic margins (C).

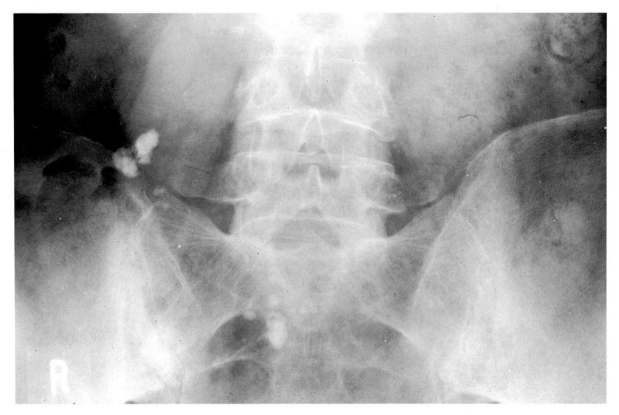

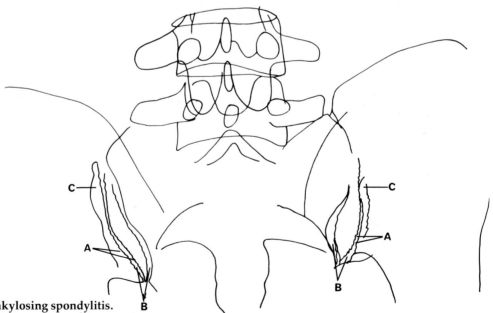

123   **Ankylosing spondylitis.**
Ankylosing spondylitis is a disease
commencing in the second and third
decades mainly in males. It involves the
intervertebral and apophyseal joints of the
spine, the costo-vertebral and
costo-transverse joints and the sacro-iliac
joints. The hips and shoulders may also be
affected.

The first example, of the sacro-iliac joints,
shows the erosive stage of the disease. The
joint margins (A) are irregular and
indistinct. The joint spaces (B) are
preserved and the adjacent bone is slightly
sclerotic (C).

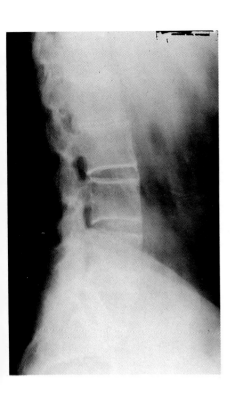
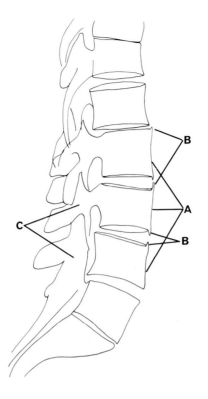

124   **Ankylosing spondylitis.**

(a)   *Lateral lumbar spine.*
There is 'squaring-off' of the anterior margins of the lumbar vertebrae (A) due to resorption of the upper and lower parts of the anterior vertebral border. There is anterior ligamentous ossification (B). The margins of the apophyseal joints (C) are ill-defined and they appear to be at least partially fused.

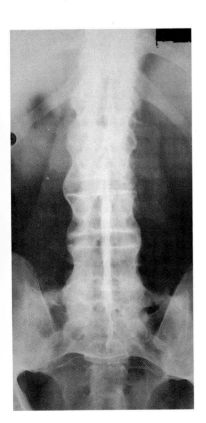
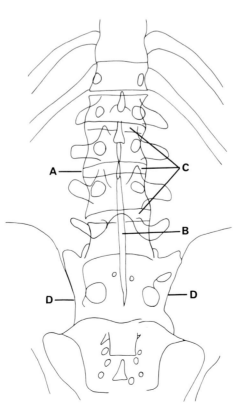

(b)   *AP view of the lumbar spine.*
There is a lateral (A) and posterior (B) ligamentous ossification causing almost complete ankylosis. The disc spaces (C) are preserved. This is the typical 'bamboo spine' of ankylosing spondylitis. The sacro-illiac joints (D) are completely ankylosed.

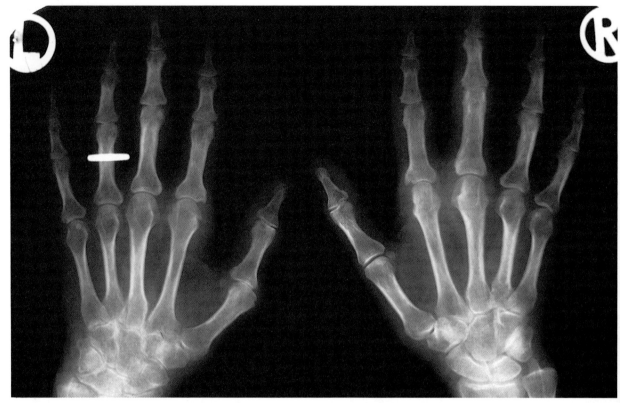

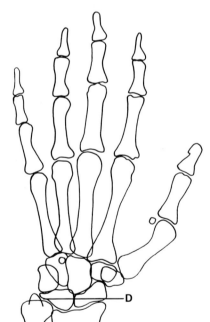

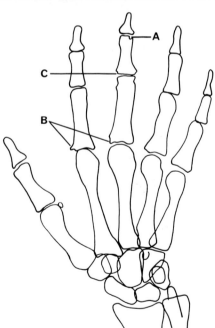

125 **Psoriatic arthropathy—hands.**
The main differences in the hands from rheumatoid arthritis are the lack of juxta-articular osteoporosis and the preference for the terminal phalangeal joints. In this case, they are narrowed and the right third middle phalangeal head is eroded (A). There are also right metacarpo-phalangeal (B) and proximal interphalangeal joint erosions (C). The left wrist joint (D) is involved.

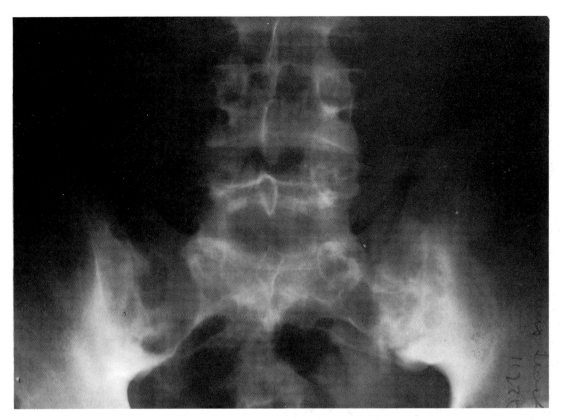

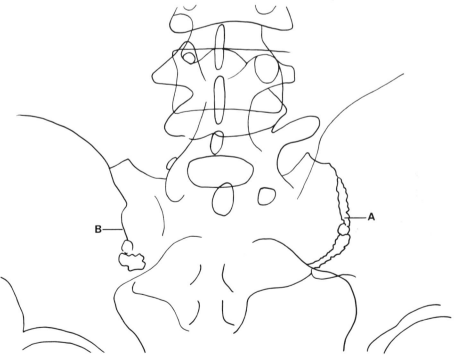

126   Psoriatic arthropathy. Sacro-iliac joints.
There is irregularity of the margins of the
left sacro-iliac joint (A) and the right joint
(B) is almost obliterated. The appearance
resembles ankylosing spondylitis.

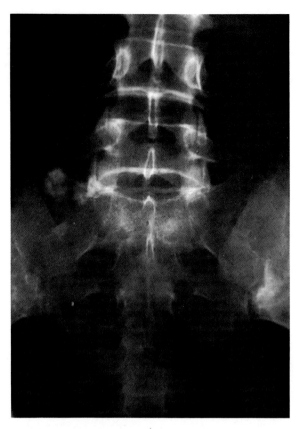

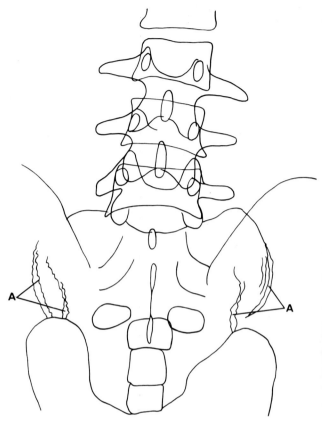

127 Reiter's disease.
Reiter's disease is a combination of arthritis, urethritis and conjunctivitis, almost always in males. It is a sexually transmitted disease but may be associated with dysentery.

(a) Sacro-iliac joints.

As in this example, the sacro-iliac joints may be involved, the appearances resembling ankylosing spondylitis. The joint margins (A) are hazy and ill-defined. It can be differentiated from ankylosing spondylitis by peripheral joint involvement and by other signs mentioned above.

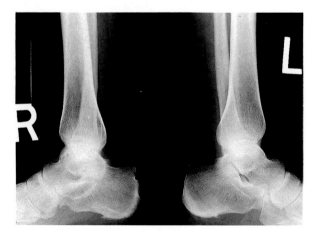

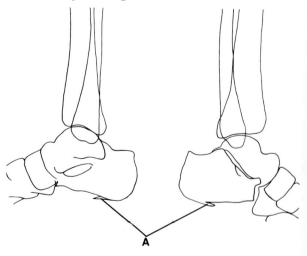

(b) Both ankles.
There are bilateral, calcaneal plantar spurs (A) due to periosteal new bone formation at

the insertions of the long plantar ligaments.

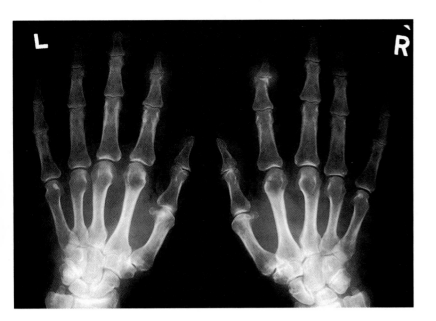

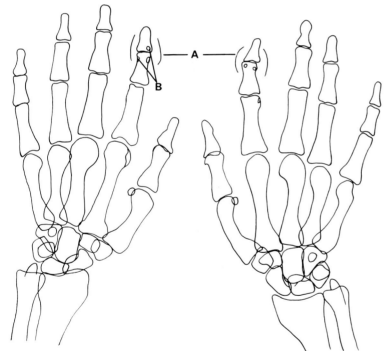

128   Gout.

In gout, the serum uric acid is elevated. The radiological changes are secondary to the deposition of urates within the synovium and secondary erosion of cartilage and bone. The classical radiological picture of calcified gouty tophi with subarticular erosions in an inflammed great toe is seldom seen nowadays. However, the toe remains the site of predilection.

In this example, in the hands, there is soft tissue swelling (A) round both second distal interphalangeal joints. 'Punched-out' subarticular erosions (B) preserving the joint surfaces are more clearly seen on the left.

In the differentiation from rheumatoid arthritis, it should be noted that, in gout, the soft tissue swelling is eccentric, the erosions are subarticular, and peri-articular osteoporosis is usually absent.

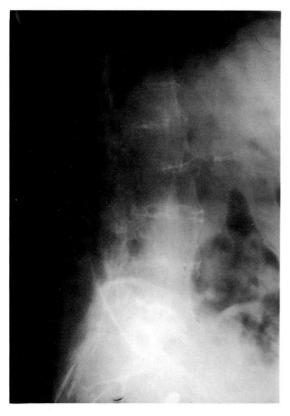

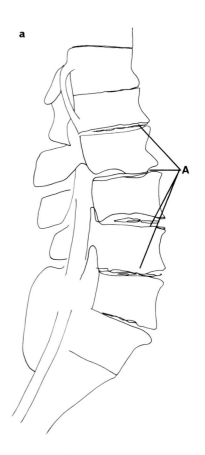

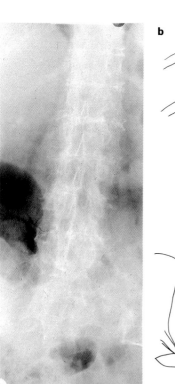

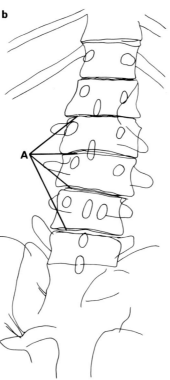

129   Alkaptonuria (ochronosis).

(a)   Lateral view of spine.

(b)   AP view of spine.
Alkaptonuria is a rare, inherited, metabolic disorder in which the deposition of homogentisic acid in the joints leads to arthropathy and articular calcification. In the spine, the disc spaces are narrowed, irregular and calcified (A).

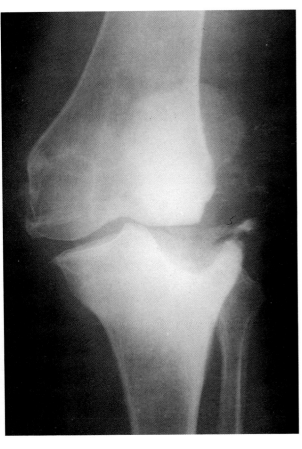

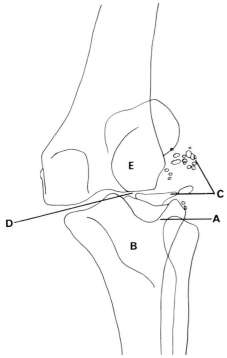

130   Neuropathic joints.
Diminution or absence of pain sense leads
to neuropathic joints. The classical
Charcot's joint of neurosyphilis is now rare.
Neuropathic joints are more commonly
found in diabetes, syringomyelia, spina
bifida and, in developing countries,
leprosy.

The first example is a typical Charcot's joint
occurring in neurosyphilis. The left knee is
involved and has a large sharply defined
defect in the lateral tibial table (A) with
sclerotic margins (B). There is
fragmentation of bone (C) in and around
the joint. The lateral femoral condyle is also
slightly flattened (D) with surrounding
sclerosis (E).

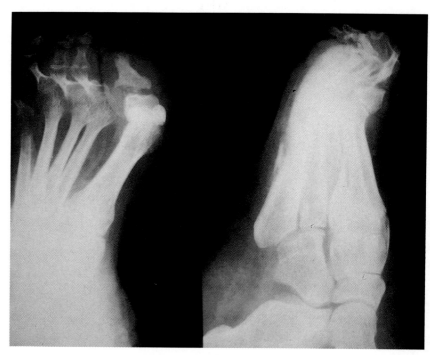

131   Diabetic arthropathy—left foot.

There is destruction of the head of the first proximal phalanx (A), the base of the first distal phalanx (B) and the head of the 5th metatarsal (C). Periosteal separation (D) is seen in the 5th metatarsal shaft.

There is also vascular calcification (E), a common finding in the diabetic foot.

The metatarso-phalangeal joints (F) are hyperextended and the proximal interphalangeal joints (G) hyperflexed as a result of diabetic neuropathy.

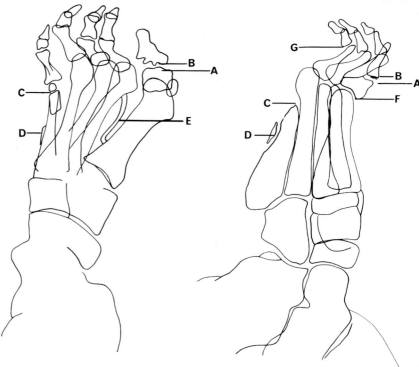

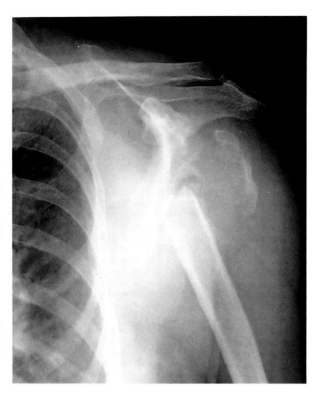
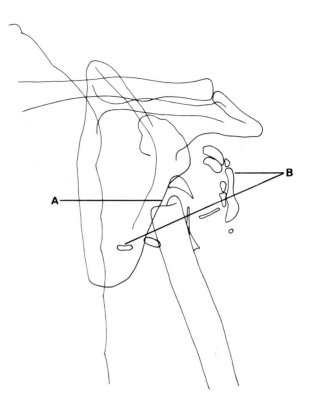

132 **Neuropathic left shoulder.**
The underlying neurological disorder is syringomyelia in which the neuropathy primarily involves the upper limbs. There is marked destruction of the proximal humerus (A) with irregular fragmentation (B).

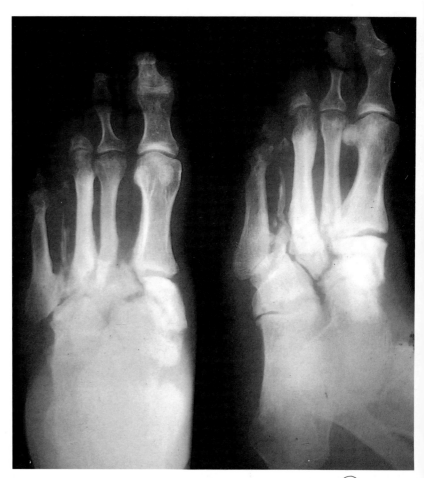

133 Neuropathic foot—leprosy.
There is loss of most of the third, fourth and fifth toes. The fourth metacarpal is narrow and tapered: the so-called 'sucked candy' appearance (A). Periosteal reaction is seen along the first metatarsal shaft (B). There is destruction of the tarsus, particularly the cuneiforms (C) with irregular tarsal joint margins (D).

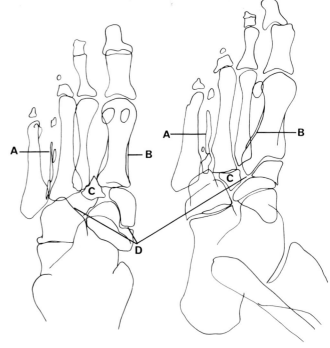

6: BONE TUMOURS

Radiological diagnosis of bone tumours can be difficult but there are a few facts which help in the differential diagnosis.

The most important of these is that bone tumours, in adults at least, are almost always secondary. Secondary tumours are usually multiple and destructive but may, for instance in prostatic carcinoma, be osteoblastic.

Primary tumours are usually solitary and often affect children and adolescents. The presence of unfused epiphyses is, therefore, important.

In general, benign tumours have much better defined margins than malignant ones. In difficult cases, close co-operation between the clinician, radiologist and pathologist is important.

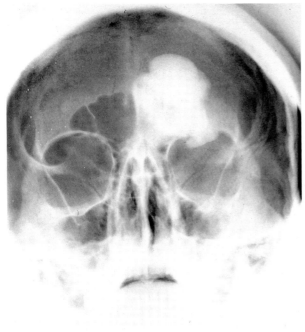

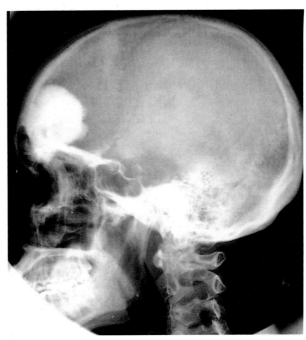

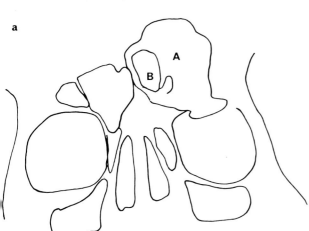

a

b

134   **Ivory osteoma of frontal sinus.**
This simple tumour arising from membranous bone is known as an ivory osteoma because of its density. It is usually a chance radiographic finding and often asymptomatic.

(a)   *PA view.*
In this example, a well-defined extremely dense tumour (A) can be seen arising from the frontal sinus (B).

(b)   *The lateral skull view of the same patient.*

163

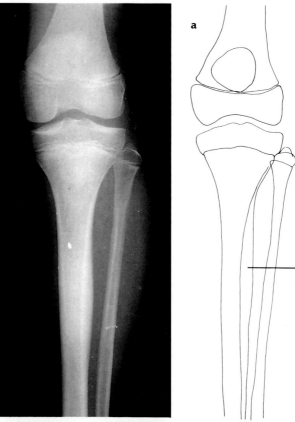

135 Osteoid osteoma.

(a) AP view of lower leg.

(b) Lateral view of lower leg. This benign, osteoid forming tumour mainly affects individuals under 30 years. It has a 2:1 male predominance. It usually affects the appendicular skeleton but may affect the axial skeleton, including the neural arches of the spine.

The most common radiological finding, seen in the tibia, is a dense sclerosis, mainly involving cortical bone (A). A small (less than 1.5 cm) lucent area in the middle of the tumour with a dense central nucleus is virtually diagnostic. However, as in this example, it may be concealed by the dense sclerosis unless tomography is done.

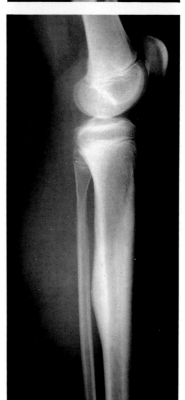

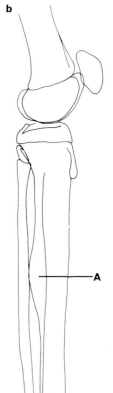

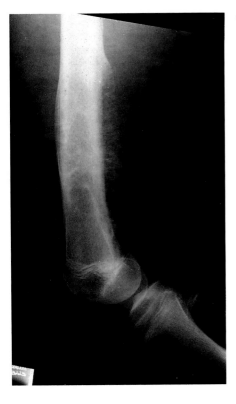
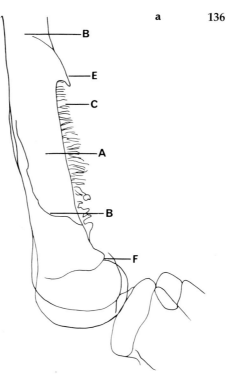

a

136 Osteosarcoma.

This is a highly malignant primary bone tumour affecting mainly the 10–25 years age-group. It can occur in older patients, usually as a complication of Paget's disease. It has a 2:1 male predominance. The tumour usually originates in the metaphysis of a long bone, most often around the knee. The radiological appearances are varied and both destruction and disorganised new bone formation can be seen. The margin of the tumour is ill-defined and there is often an associated soft tissue shadow. New bone tumour formation may be seen within the shadow. Periosteal destruction and reaction are common.

(a) Expansile lesion in the distal femur.

An expansile lesion (A) with ill-defined margins (B). New bone formation is seen postero-medially in the soft tissues (C) in the form of 'sun-ray' spiculation. There is also periosteal reaction (D) on the opposite side of the bone, showing that the tumour goes all the way through the shaft. There is periosteal elevation, known as 'Codman's triangle' at the proximal end of the tumour (E). It should be noted that this is a young patient as the epiphyses have not fused. The tumour does not cross the distal femoral epiphyseal line (F).

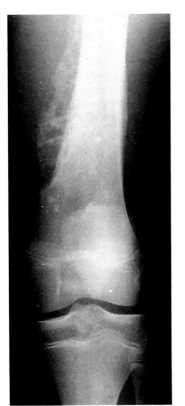
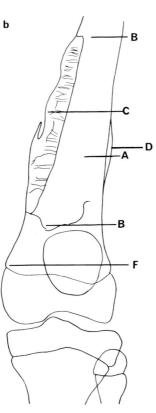

b

(b) Lateral view of the same patient.

165

137   Osteosarcoma.

(a) *Osteosarcoma of the fibula.*
     There is very dense
     periosteal and new bone
     formation (A).
     This variety, arising in
     the cortex, is sometimes
     known as parosteal
     sarcoma.

(b) *Lateral view of the same
     patient.*

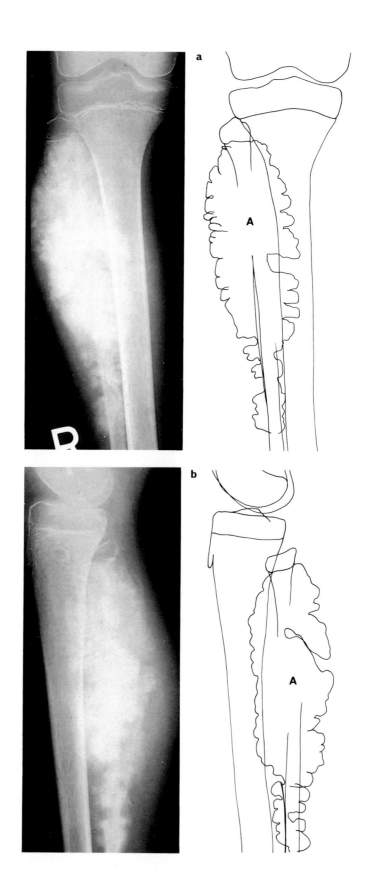

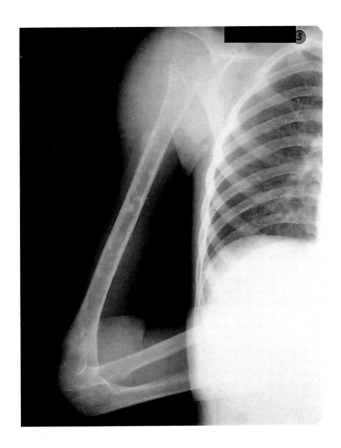

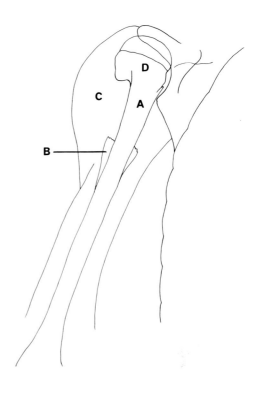

138 **Osteosarcoma of the upper humerus.**
This is a destructive upper humeral tumour (A). Its inferior margin is so poorly defined that it is not possible to tell where it is. Virtually the whole humeral shaft appears abnormal. Well-defined 'Codman's triangles' (B) are present. There is marked soft tissue swelling (C). There is a pathological fracture of the humeral neck (D).

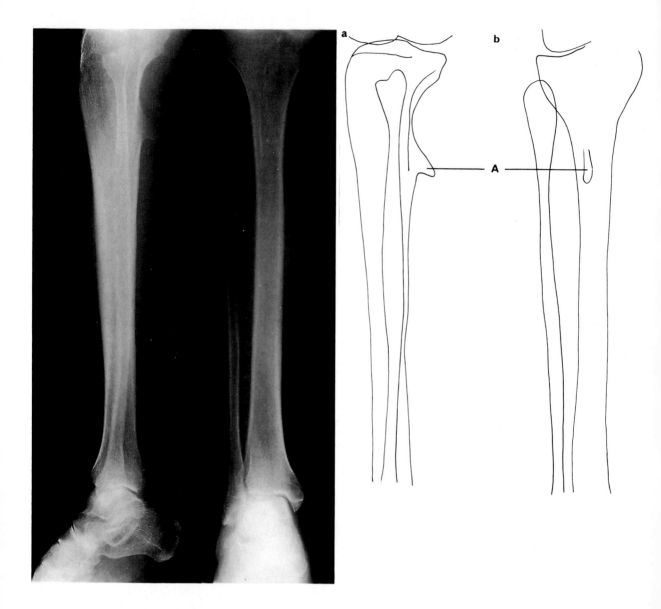

139   Exostosis of the upper tibia.

(a) *Lateral view.*
There is a simple bony protuberance arising from the posterior aspect of the upper tibia (A) seen in profile in the lateral view. If such a lesion is cartilage-capped, it is called an osteochondroma. The cartilage cap can only be seen if it calcifies.

(b) *The AP view of the same patient.*
The osteoma is seen 'en face' and is barely visible (A).

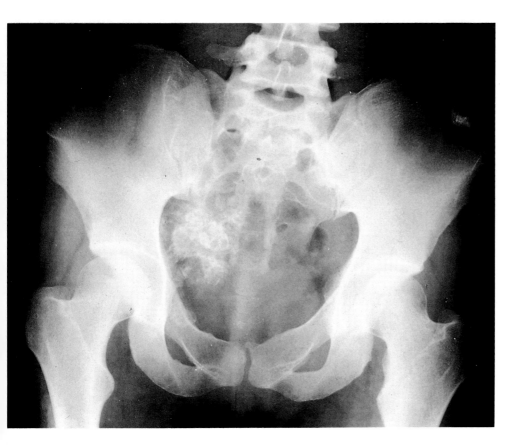

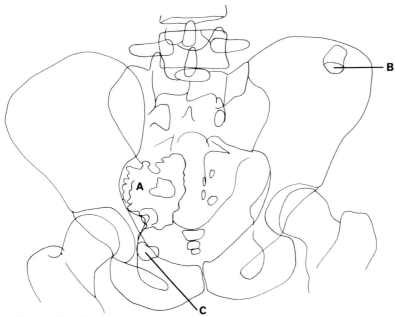

140 Sacral osteochondroma.
There is florid calcification (A) of the cartilage cap of the enchondroma. Despite its irregular, expansile appearance, it is a benign tumour. Other smaller osteochondromata are seen arising from the left ilium (B) and right ischium (C).

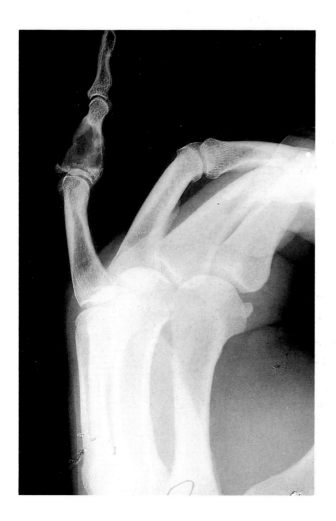

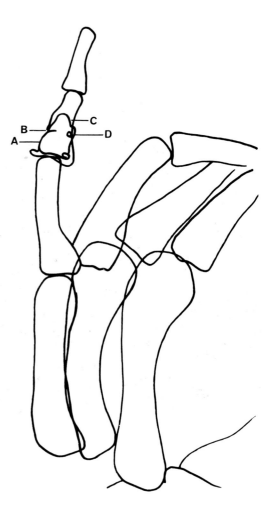

141 **Enchondroma of the fifth proximal phalanx.**

This is a benign, expansile bone tumour, often found in digits. The cortex is thinned (A) and there is a pathological fracture (B). The tumour margin (C) is slightly scalloped. Faint flecks of calcification (D) can be seen within the tumour. These are caused by calcifying cartilage and virtually confirm the diagnosis.

142 **Multiple enchondromatosis—Ollier's ▶ disease.**

This could be classified under the heading of congenital or developmental bone disease as dyschondroplasia. In this example, multiple expansile tumours (A) are seen in the metacarpals and phalanges. The appearances are the same as in the single enchondroma (see **141**) and calcification is a helpful feature. However, in this case it is not obvious. Unlike the solitary form, these tumours may undergo chondrosarcomatous change. If accompanied by cavernous haemangiomata (Mafucci's syndrome), malignant transformation is more likely (see Congenital Abnormalities).

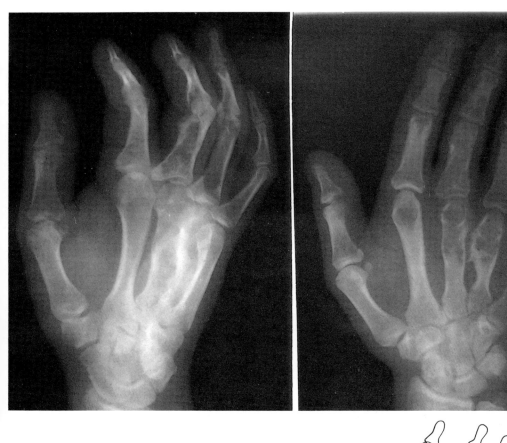

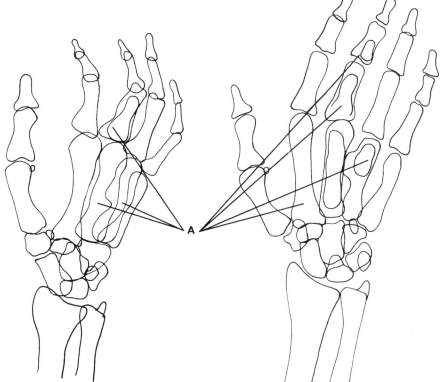

143   Non-ossifying fibroma (fibrous cortical defect).

(a)   *AP view.*
This is a benign lesion usually found incidentally in children, adolescents or young adults. This example in the distal femur, a common site, shows the salient features. It has a subcortical situation with a well-defined margin (A), a radiolucent centre with loculation (B) and slight cortical expansion (C).

(b)   *The lateral view of the same patient.*

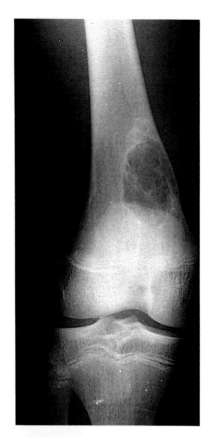
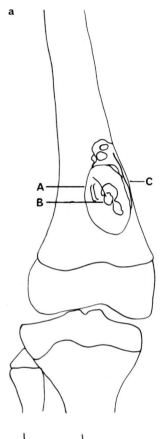

a

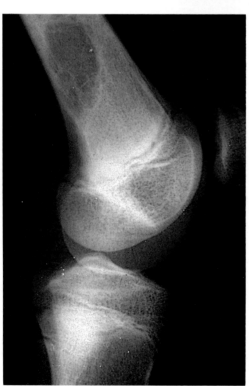
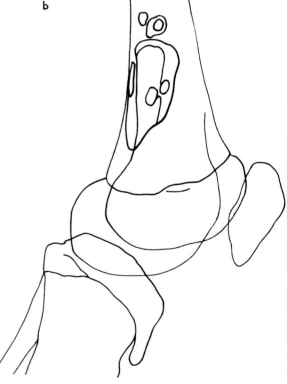

b

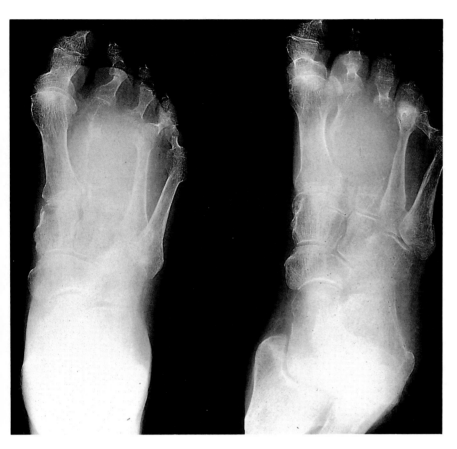

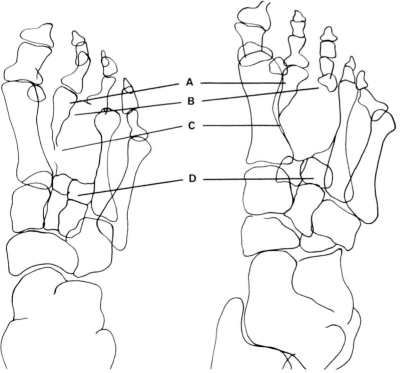

144 **Fibrosarcoma.**
This malignant tumour
is arising from either the
2nd (A) or the 3rd (B)
metatarsal and is
destroying both. It is
eroding cortex (C) and
has ill-defined margins
(D). The radiological
appearances are those of
a malignant tumour
arising in bone or in
adjacent soft tissue.
Biopsy is required for
diagnosis.

173

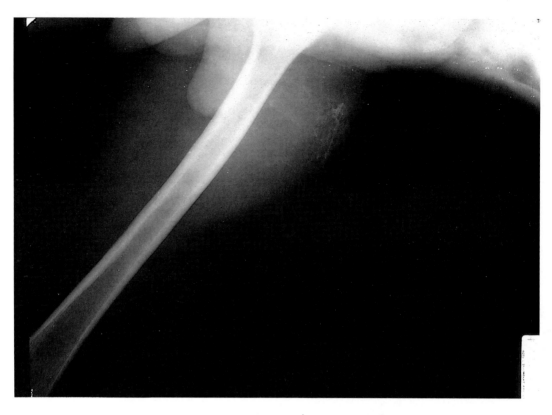

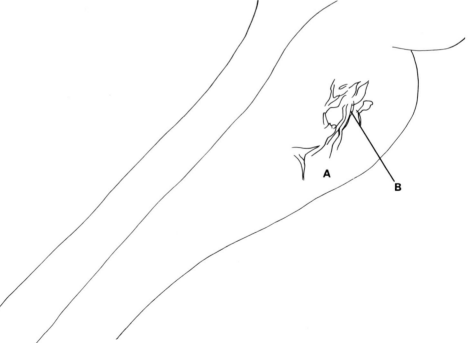

145   Spindle cell sarcoma of thigh.
This sarcoma is arising in soft tissue rather than in bone. There is soft tissue swelling (A) and irregular ossification within the mass (B). The appearances are not specific and biopsy is required for diagnosis.

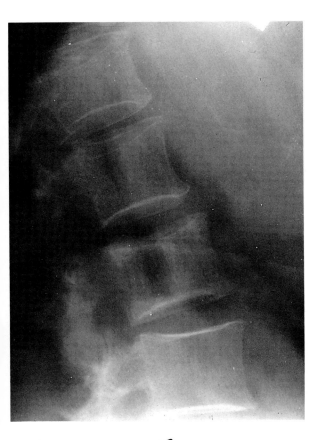

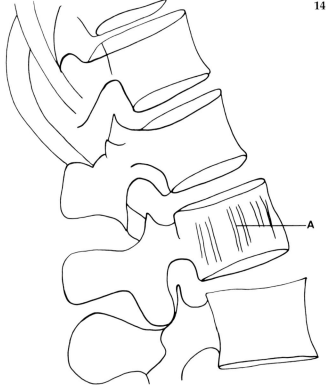

146 **Solitary haemangioma of a lumbar vertebra.**
This benign tumour has a characteristic appearance in the spine. The vertebral body has a striated appearance (A). It is not expanded. Compression fractures occur rarely.

A

147 Haemangioma of skull.

(a) *PA view.*

(b) *Lateral view.*
The appearance in the skull is different from that in the vertebra but is still characteristic. A lucent tumour (A) with well-defined margins (B) containing central radiating 'sun-burst' or 'spoked-wheel' densities (C) is typical.

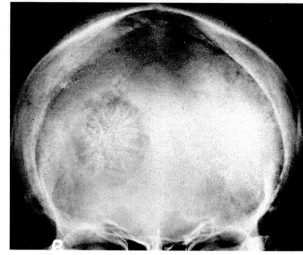

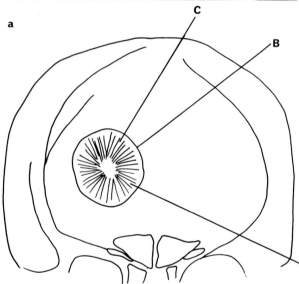

a

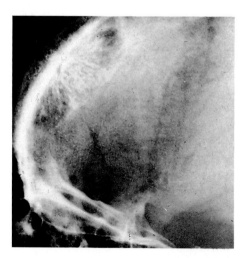

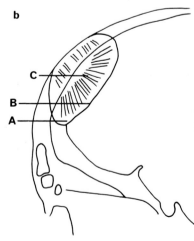

b

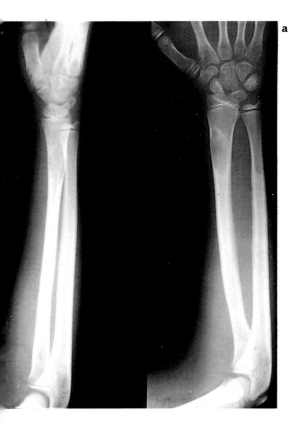
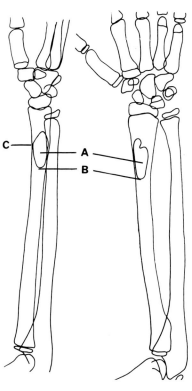

a

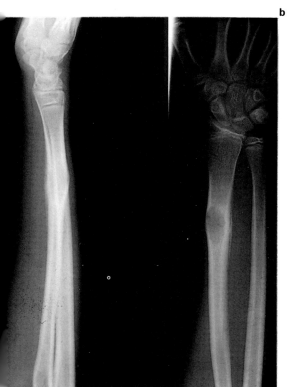
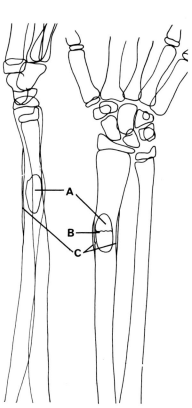

b

148   Simple bone cyst.

(a)   *Simple bone cyst of radius.* There is a benign radiolucent cyst (A) with a well-defined margin (B) in the distal radial diaphysis. The radius is slightly expanded (C). A simple cyst may be a chance radiological finding but may be painful or undergo spontaneous fracture.

(b)   *The same patient, three and a half years later.* The cyst (A) appears to have migrated proximally in the diaphysis. This is because of normal metaphyseal bone growth distal to it. Such apparent 'migration' is a feature of simple bone cyst. There is now a pathological fracture (B) with associated periosteal reaction (C).

177

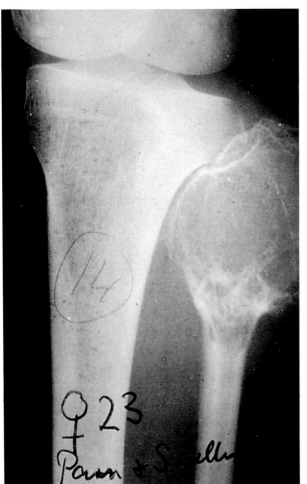
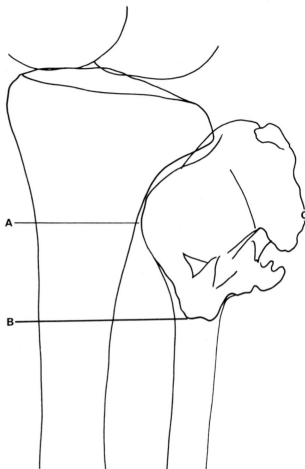

149   **Aneurysmal bone cyst of fibula.**
This a benign bone tumour which causes considerable expansion and thinning of bone (A). Its margin is usually well-defined (B) but, in this case, its lateral margin is poorly defined with cortical destruction (C). In this example, the epiphyses have fused but more usually the tumour occurs before epiphyseal fusion. However, it can occur in the third decade. If the epiphysis is unfused, this is a useful differentiating feature from giant cell tumour which occurs after epiphyseal closure.

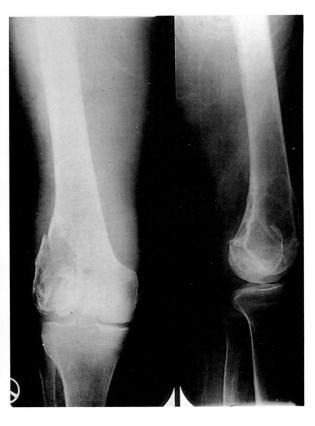
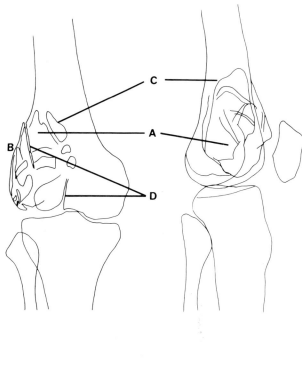

150   Giant cell tumour of distal femur.
This is a tumour of low-grade malignancy which occurs in young to middle-aged adults after epiphyseal closure. It has a subarticular, eccentric situation at the bone end. It is osteolytic (A) expansile and the cortex is thinned (B). The endosteal margin (C) is less clear-cut than in purely benign tumours. As in this case, a pathological fracture (D) may occur.

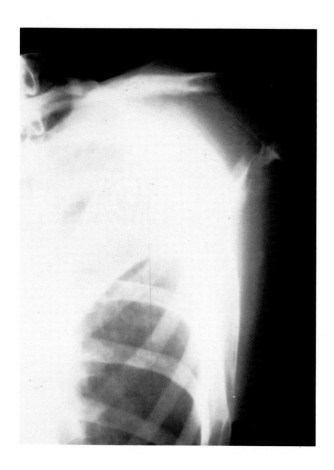

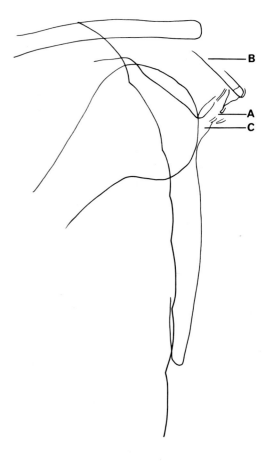

151   Ewing's tumour.
This is a malignant round cell tumour, usually occurring in the second decade. It is destructive and has no specific features. It may mimic other malignant bone tumours and osteomyelitis. Periosteal reaction is common.

This example, in the scapula, shows bony destruction of the scapular spine (A) and virtual disappearance of the acromion (B). The tumour margin (C) is poorly defined.

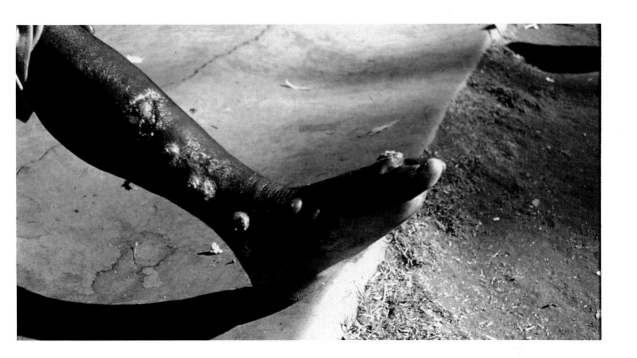

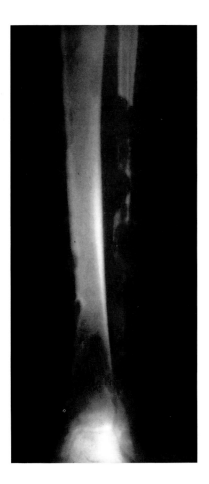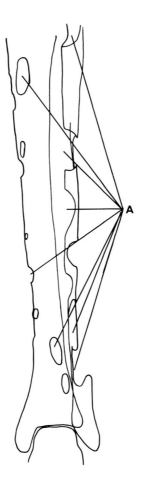

152   Kaposi's sarcoma.
There are multiple soft
tissue tumours which
eventually erode bone.
It is relatively common
in Africa but until
recently has been rare in
Europeans. However, it
is one of the tumours
which occur in AIDS.

*(a)   A clinical example of the
soft tissue tumours.*

*(b)   X-ray—the tibia and fibula
of a different patient.*
There are multiple,
'punched-out' lesions of
the tibia and fibula (A)
giving rise to a 'moth-
eaten' appearance.

181

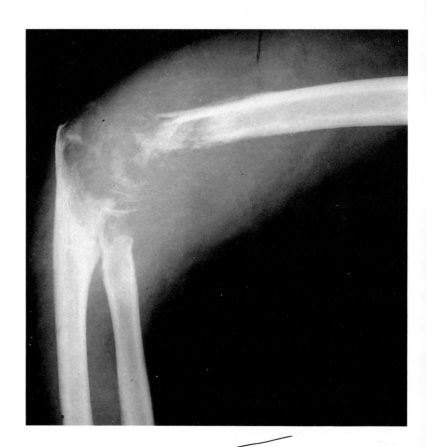

153 Synovioma of the left elbow.
This malignant tumour of the joint capsule causes marked soft tissue swelling (A) and irregular destruction of the bones on both sides of the joint (B). Calcification occurs but is not marked in this example.

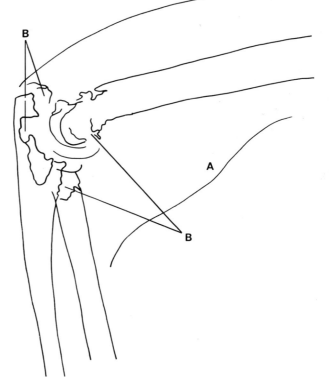

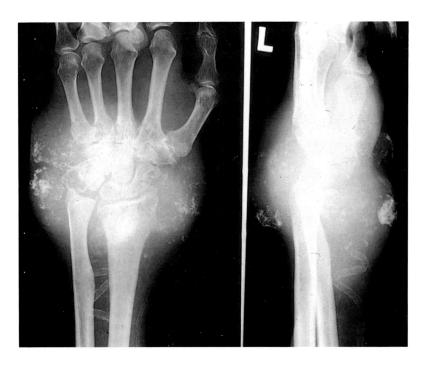

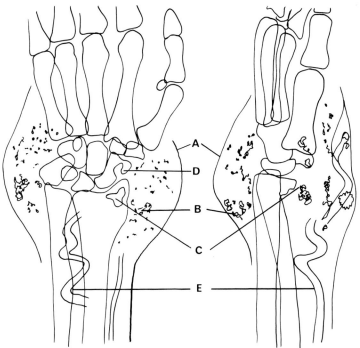

154   Synovioma of wrist and carpus.
This example, in a different patient, shows massive soft tissue swelling (A) and marked, irregular calcification (B). Bone destruction is less marked but is seen in the distal radius (C) and scaphoid (D). The serpiginous vascular calcification is unrelated (E).

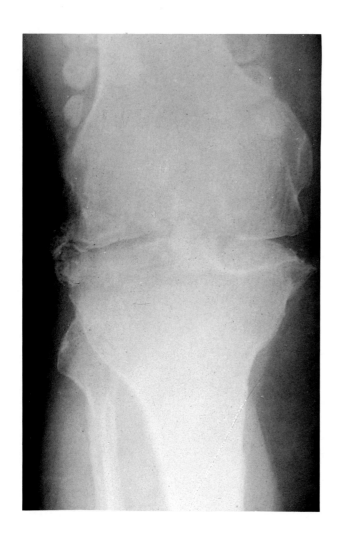

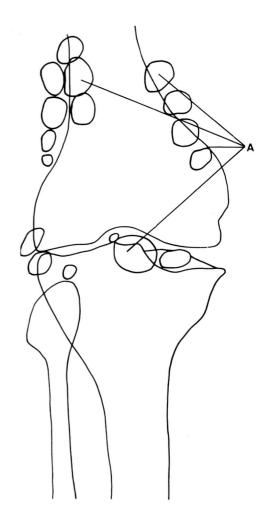

155   Osteochondromatosis.

(a) PA view.

184

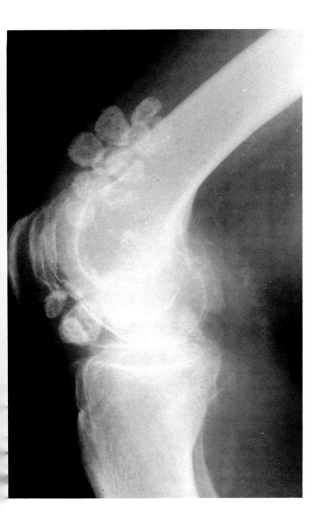
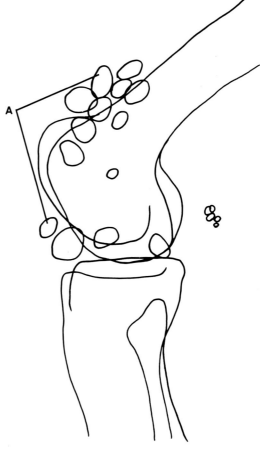

(b) *Lateral view.*

Multiple, ossified cartilaginous masses (A) are seen arising from the synovium of the knee joint capsule. They may lead to secondary degenerative change.

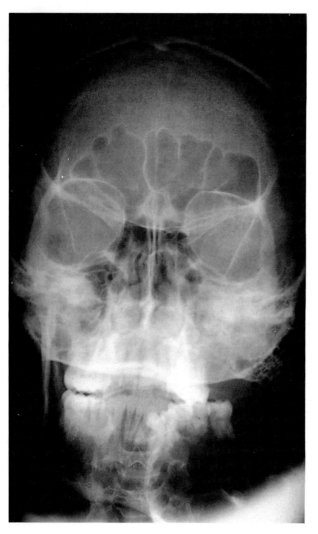

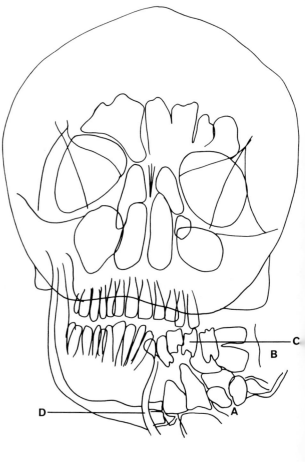

156   Ameloblastoma of mandible.
This is a locally malignant tumour which
very rarely metastasises. It is more common
in Africans than in Europeans.

(a)   The AP view of skull and mandible.
A huge, expansile tumour can be seen
arising from the left mandible. The tumour
has a scalloped appearance (A). The outer
margin (B) is so thin that it cannot be seen.
The teeth (C) are displaced. The tumour
does not cross the mid-line (D).

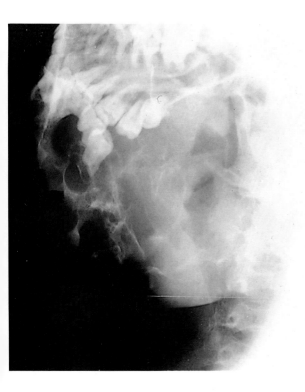
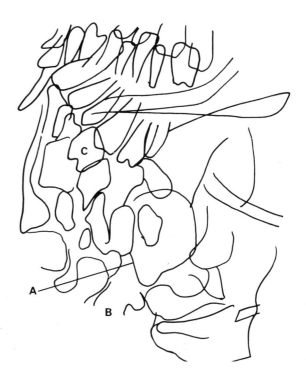

(b)   *Oblique view of mandible in the same patient.*
The scalloped appearance of the tumour
(A), the poorly defined outer margin (B)
and the displaced teeth (C) are more clearly
seen.

157   Metastatic carcinoma.
Metastatic bone carcinoma is much more common than primary bone tumour. Metastatic deposits are usually multiple and destructive. They may also be osteolytic or mixed.

(a)   *Metastasis of right femur.*
This is an example of a solitary metastatic deposit, in this case from bronchial carcinoma. There is a large, fairly well-defined destructive tumour (A) with no evidence of marginal sclerosis.

(b)   *AP view.*
It can be seen clearly that the cortex (A) is breached and that the mass extends to soft tissue (B).

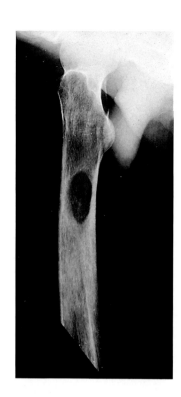

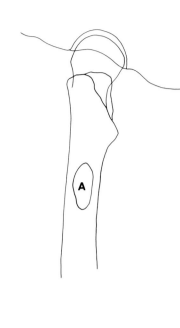
a

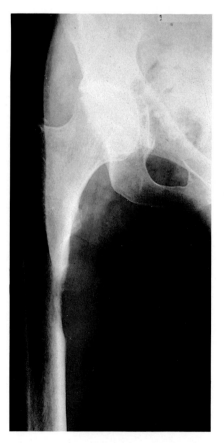

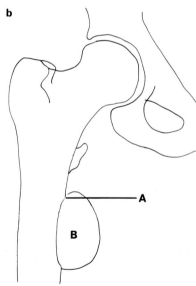
b

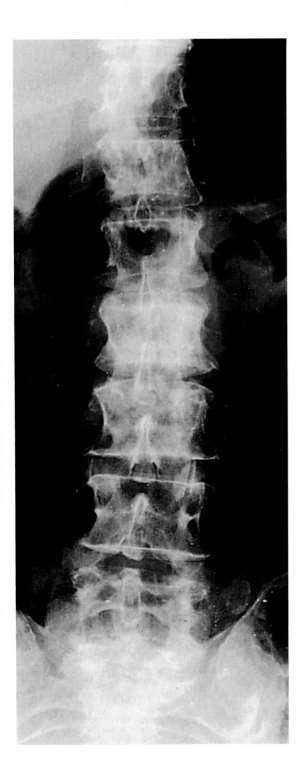

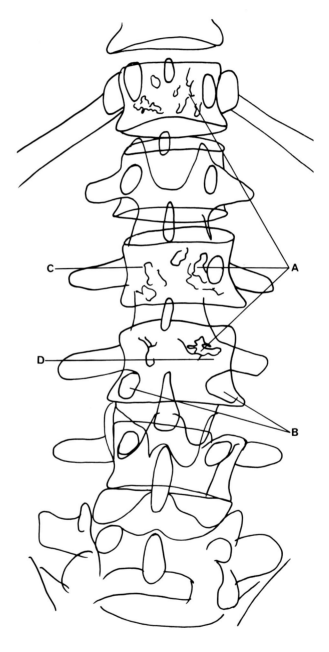

158 **Mixed osteoblastic and osteolytic metastases from breast carcinoma.**
The bone texture of DV12, LV2 and LV3 is altered. There is an irregular sclerotic pattern (A) in all three vertebrae and lytic areas are seen in LV3 (B). The right pedicle of LV2 is absent (C) and both pedicles of LV3 are ill-defined (D). The absence of pedicles differentiates this from myeloma.

159   Osteoblastic metastases from prostatic carcinoma.

(a) *Lateral view.*
Dense, osteoblastic metastatic disease almost replaces the normal bone pattern in the lumbar, sacral and lower dorsal spine, pelvis and lower ribs.

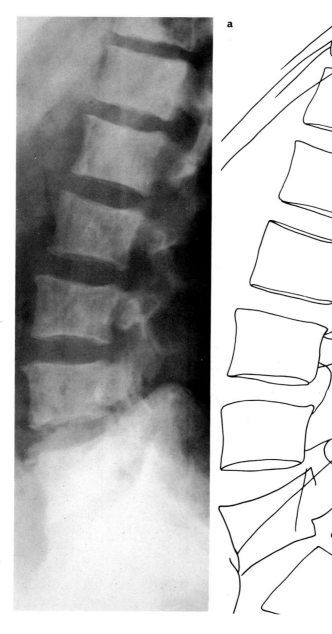

a

(b) *Pelvis and proximal femora of the same patient.*
Confluent, osteoblastic metastases completely replace the normal pelvic bony trabecular pattern. More discrete osteoblastic metastases are seen in the proximal femora (A).
These appearances can be differentiated from Paget's disease by the lack of bone expansion, by the absence of bony secondary to softening and by the absence of any signs of the spongy form of Paget's disease.

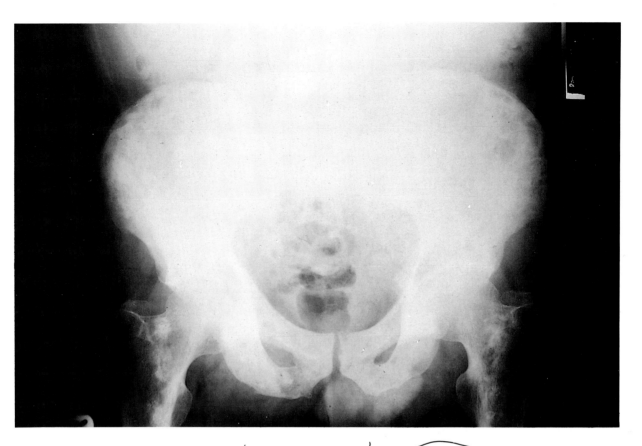

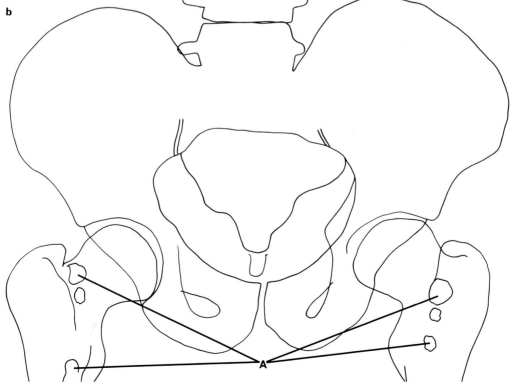

b

191

7: BONE CHANGES IN THE RETICULOSES AND HAEMOPOIETIC DISORDERS

Bone changes in the reticuloses may be difficult to differentiate from bone tumours. Usually the bony abnormalities are seen in patients with a known reticulosis but, occasionally, the disease first manifests itself as an osseous lesion.

In haemopoietic disorders, when bone changes occur, they are due to marrow hypertrophy, replacement of marrow by abnormal tissue and consequent abnormal bone modelling. Frank bone destruction may occur in the aggressive disorders such as leukaemia.

Other features include an abnormal trabecular pattern and bone infarction.

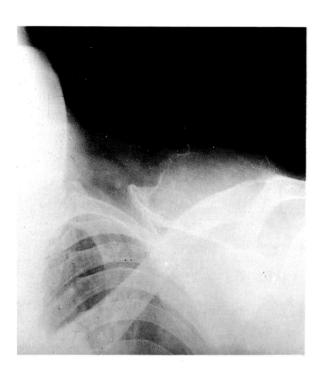
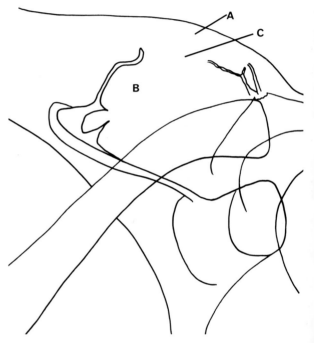

160   **Plasmacytoma.**
Plasmacytoma is the solitary form of multiple myeloma. This example, in the scapula, shows marked soft tissue swelling (A), bone expansion (B) and thinning of the cortex which has been breached (C).

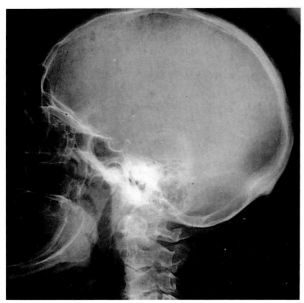

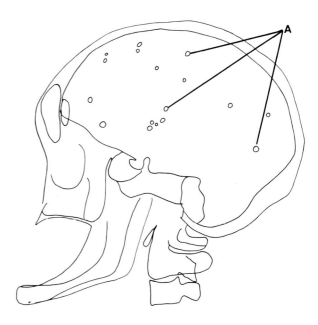

161 **Multiple myeloma.**
Multiple myeloma is much more common than plasmacytoma. Its main differential diagnoses are from multiple metastases and osteoporosis. In the early stages, it can be difficult to differentiate from the latter on radiological grounds alone.

(a) *Myeloma of skull.*
There are multiple, characteristic, round, osteolytic lesions (A) without sclerotic borders in the vault.

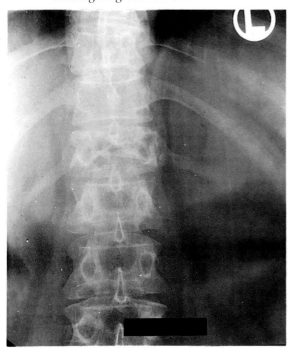

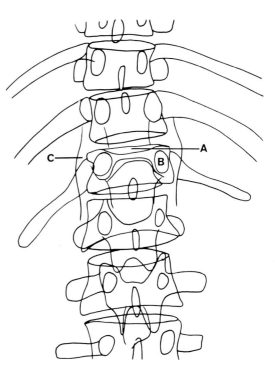

(b) *Myeloma of DV12 in the same patient.*
There is collapse of the vertebral body (A). The pedicles (B) are intact, a useful differentiating point from metastatic carcinoma. There is also a little

paravertebral tissue swelling (C). This is more likely to occur in myeloma than in metastases but it is not particularly marked in this example.

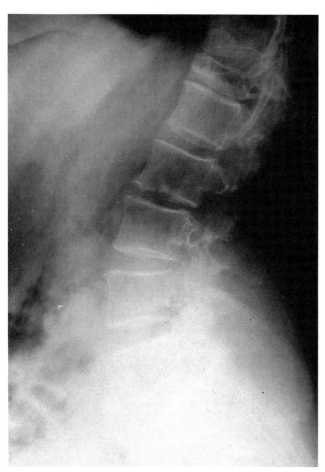

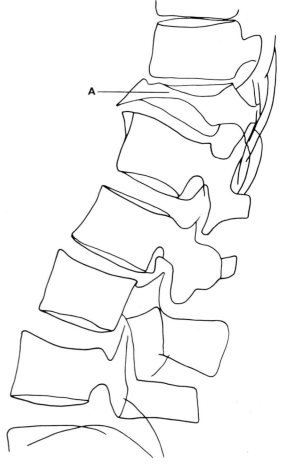

(c) *Myeloma of DV12.*
Lateral view—showing collapse of the
vertebral body (A).

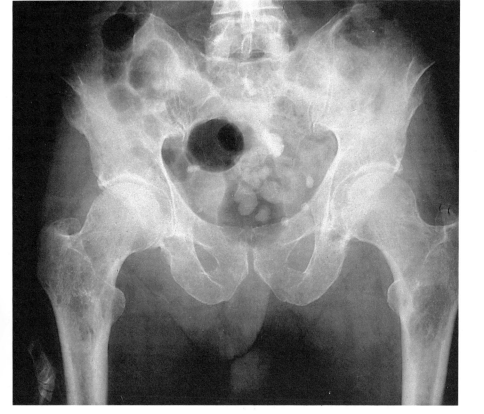

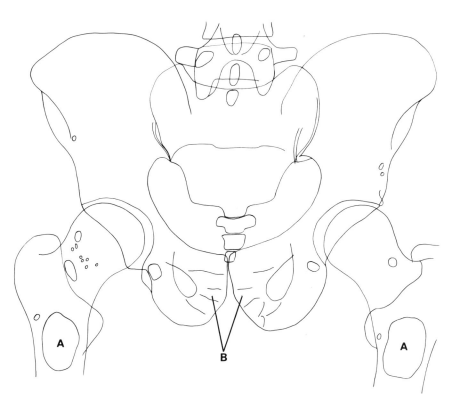

162 Myeloma of the pelvis and femora in a different patient.
There are multiple lucent defects of different sizes, the ones in the upper femora being particularly large (A). There is also a generalised alteration in bone texture. The pubic bones on both sides are particularly radiolucent (B).

195

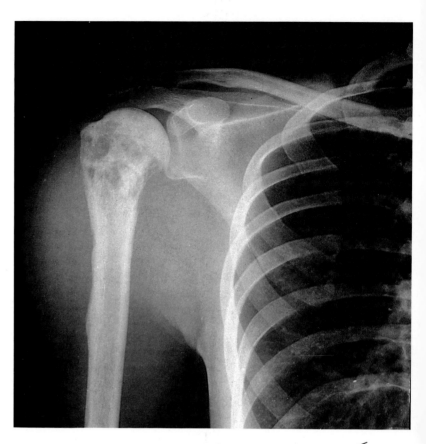

163 Hodgkin's disease.
There is a mixed lytic (A) and sclerotic (B) lesion in the upper humerus. Another lytic area (C) is seen eroding cortex. There is nothing specific about the appearances. Hodgkin's disease had been diagnosed from a cervical node biopsy. When the reticuloses involve bone, radiological differentiation from secondary or primary tumours may be difficult. Diagnosis is easier when the patient is known to have a lymphoma. Occasionally, however, the bone lesion will be seen before other manifestations.

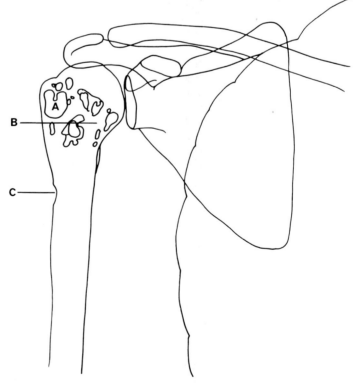

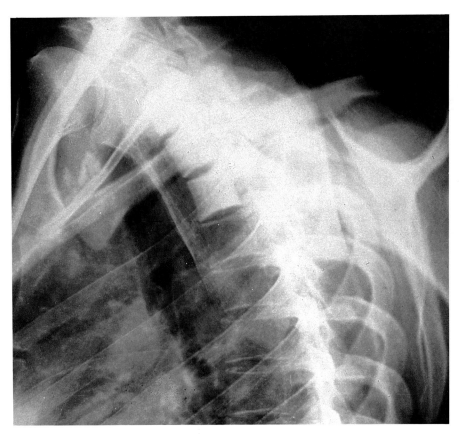

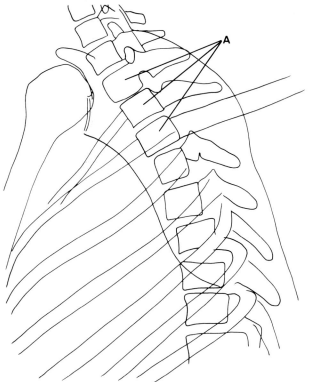

164 **Hodgkin's disease of the upper dorsal vertebrae.**
DV1, 2 and 3 are dense (A) due to the presence of osteoblastic disease. Such spinal lesions may be found incidentally in X-rays of chest and abdomen, and lead to investigation for evidence of lymphoma elsewhere.

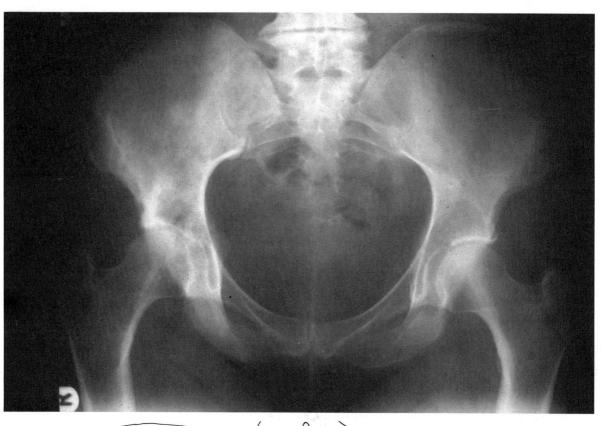

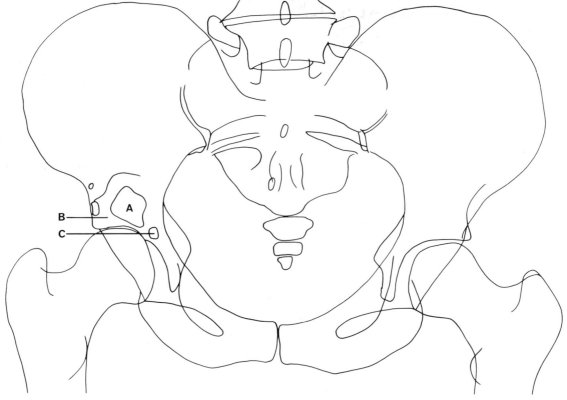

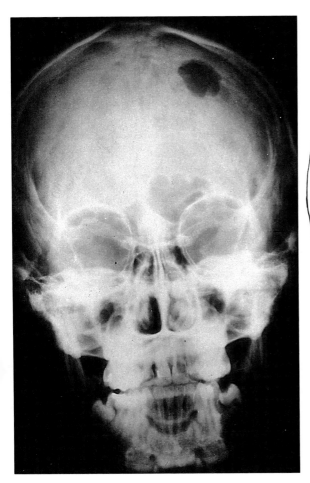

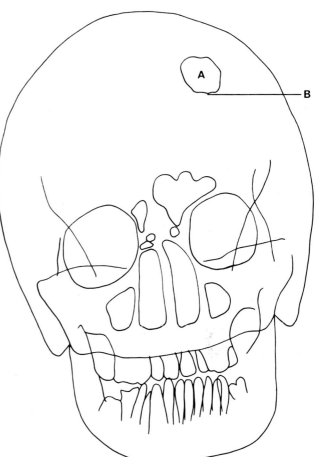

166 **Eosinophilic granuloma of the skull.**
There is a well-defined, lucent defect (A) in
the skull with a clear-cut margin (B). When
such tumours are solitary, they are usually
called eosinophilic granuloma. However,
eosinophilic granuloma is the benign end of
a group of reticuloendothelioses, generally
known as 'Histiocytosis-X'. The group
comprises, in order of increasing
malignancy: eosinophilic granuloma,
Hand-Schuller-Christian disease and
Letterer-Siwe disease.

165 **Non-Hodgkin's lymphoma of pelvis.**
◄ There is a large, lucent lytic area (A) in the
ilium, just above the acetabulum. Its
margins are ill-defined but there is some
sclerosis laterally (B). Other, smaller
radiolucent defects are present also (C).

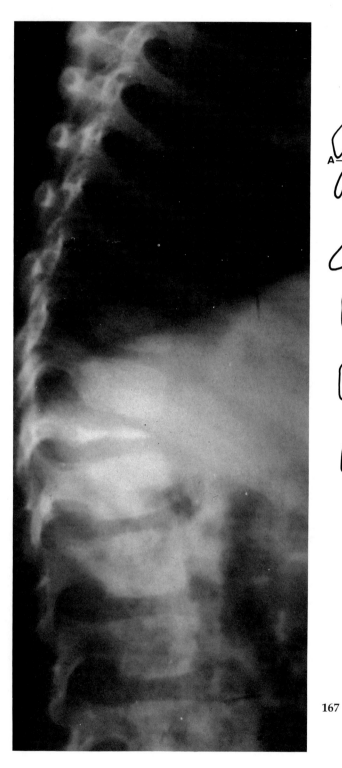

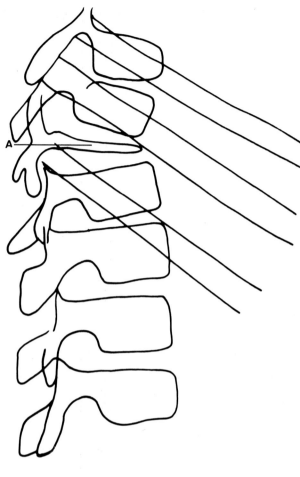

167 **Eosinophilic granuloma of DV12.**
Eosinophilic granuloma is one cause of the
solitary, dense, flat vertebra (A) (vertebra
plana).

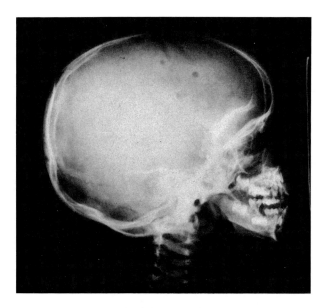

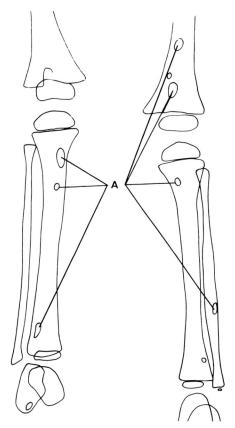

168 **Hand-Schuller-Christian disease.**
This variant of Histiocytosis-X occurs in
children and adolescents.

(a) Skull—lateral view.
Three small, well-defined lucent defects can
be seen (A).

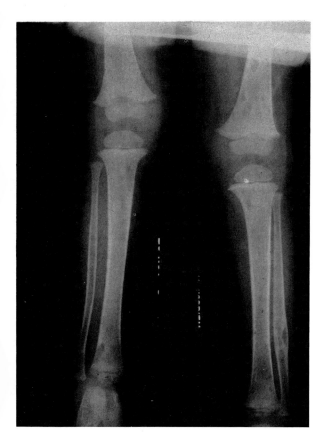

(b) Both tibiae and fibulae of the same patient.
Multiple, well-defined, lucent lesions are
shown.

169   Gaucher's disease.
The skeletal manifestations of this disease which typically, but not exclusively, affects young Jewish females, are due to deposits of lipid-laden histiocytes in the marrow. This leads to osteoporosis, expansion of the marrow cavity and bone infarcts.

(a) *Distal femur.*
In this example, there is gross widening of the femur with loss of medullary bone pattern (A) and dense sclerotic bands (B). The irregular, sclerotic appearance of bone infarction (C) can be seen in the tibia.

(b) *Proximal femur.*
The upper femoral shaft is involved although it is not as wide as the lower. There is partial collapse of the femoral head (A), due to avascular necrosis. Secondary osteoarthritis is present with sclerosis and osteophyte formation (B).

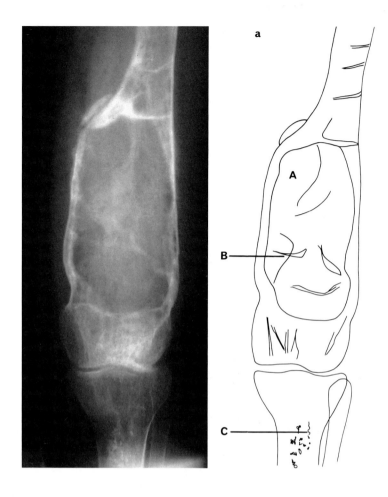

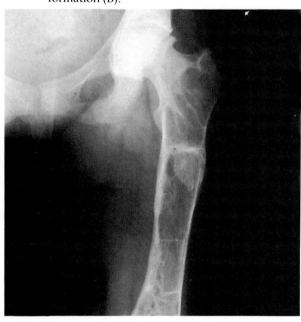

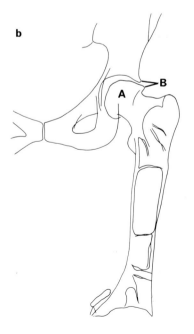

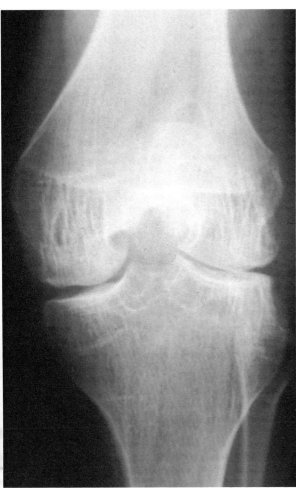

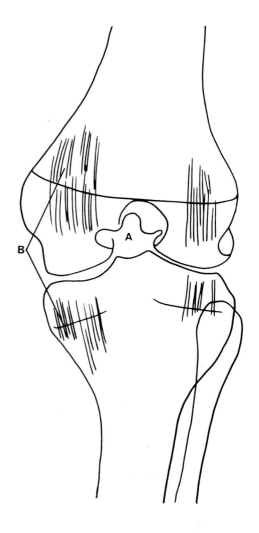

170   Haemophilia.
The joint changes in haemophilia are secondary to recurrent intra-articular haemorrhages. This view of the knee shows the classical appearance of widening and deepening of the intercondylar notch of the femur (A) secondary to haemorrhage into the insertions of cruciate ligaments. The bones are generally osteopaenic but with a few sclerotic trabeculae, giving rise to a striated appearance (B).

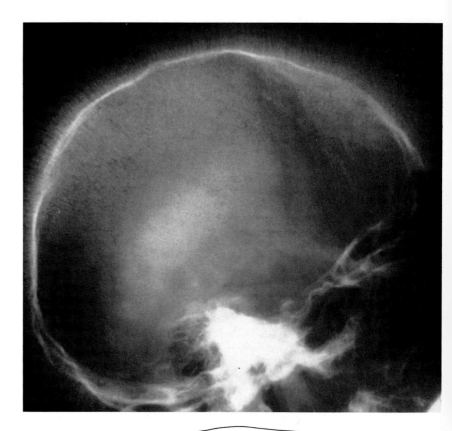

171 Thalassaemia major.
The bone changes in
thalassaemia major are
due to marrow
hyperplasia expanding
the medulla. The bone
trabeculae are widely
separated, coarse and
dense. This lateral skull
view shows the classical
'hair-on-end'
appearance (A)
associated with marked
increased width of the
skull bones (B).
However, this
appearance is by no
means always present.

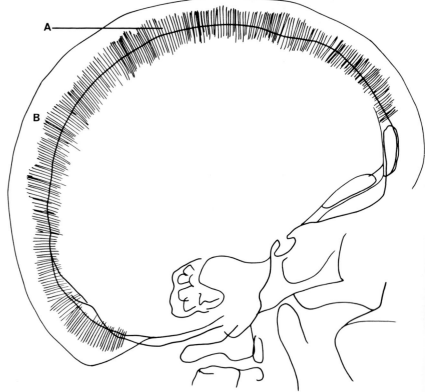

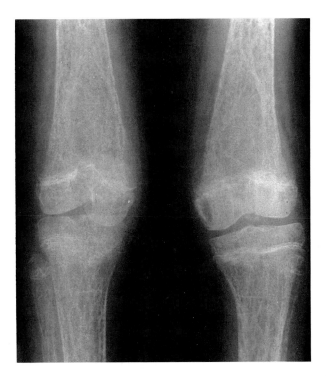
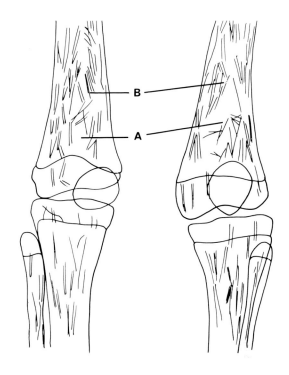

172   Thalassaemia major in a different patient.

(a) *Both knees.*
Both distal femora are expanded with a tendency to be 'flask-shaped'. The bones are generally osteopaenic (A) with a sparse, coarse, dense trabecular pattern (B).

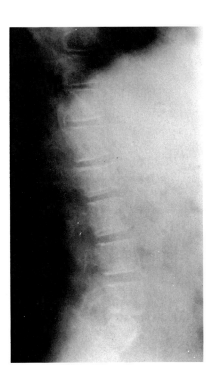
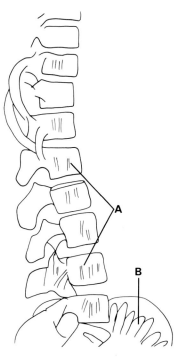

(b) *Lateral lumbo-sacral spine.*
The vertebral bodies are slightly expanded and are osteopaenic. A few coarse trabeculae are seen (A). These are more marked in the ilium (B).

(c) *Chest.*
The ribs are expanded with a sparse, coarse trabecular pattern (A). There is cardiomegaly (B) secondary to anaemia.

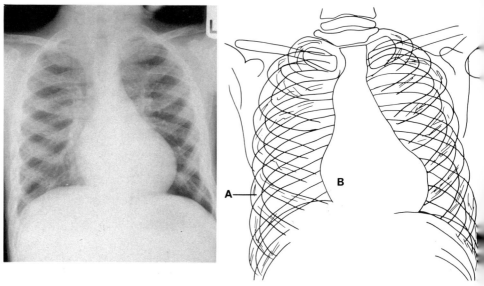

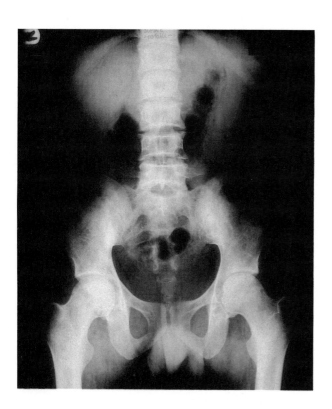

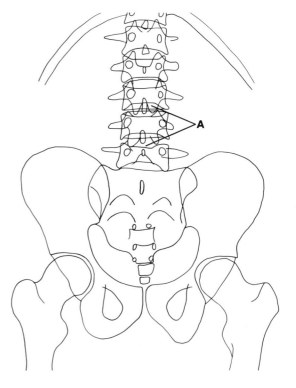

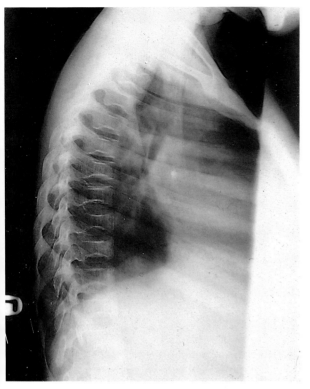

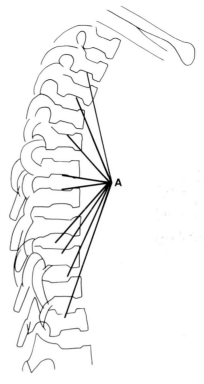

174 **Haemoglobin SO disease.**
In this lateral view of the thoracic spine, flattening of the vertebral end plates (A) is clearly seen. This appearance has been described erroneously as 'cod-fish' vertebrae. It can be seen that it is the disc spaces and not the vertebrae which are fish-shaped. (Illustration reproduced from A.G. Kendall and J.F. Calder: Radiological Changes in Haemoglobin SO disease *East African Medical Journal* 56, 7, 1979, by permission of the Editor.)

173 **Sickle cell anaemia.**
◄ Although marrow hyperlasia does occur in sickle cell anaemia, it is not so obvious radiologically as in thalassaemia. In children, the bones may appear a little osteoporotic and in adults, as in this case, a diffusely increased trabecular pattern may develop. Bone infarction is the most striking radiological appearance in sickle cell disease. This affects epiphyses particularly, especially of the proximal femur. In this example, there is flattening of the vertebral end plates (A). These end plates are the secondary centres of ossification of the vertebral bones and are, therefore, analogous to the epiphyses of long bones.

Classical homozygous sickle cell anaemia may be designated haemoglobin SS disease. Combinations of abnormal haemoglobins may occur, e.g. haemoglobins SC, SD and SO. The clinical manifestations of these combinations may be less severe but the radiological appearances are similar. The example illustrated is from a patient with haemoglobin SC disease.

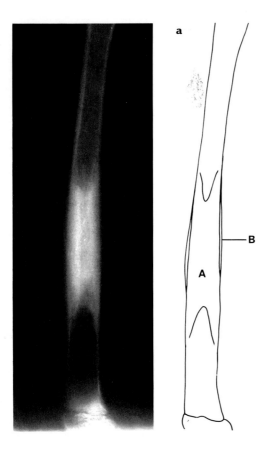

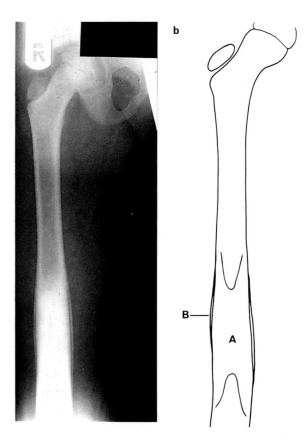

175   Sickle cell (Hb SS) disease of the femur with complicating osteomyelitis.
There is a well-demarcated dense, slightly expansile area (A) in the distal femur with associated periosteal reaction (B). Unless breakdown of bone has taken place, it can be difficult to distinguish between a bone infarct and osteomyelitis on radiological grounds alone. The presence of periosteal reaction suggests osteomyelitis but it can also occur in uncomplicated infarction. This lesion subsequently broke down and staphylococci were isolated from it.
The presence of osteomyelitis, especially if it is multifocal, should make one suspect sickle cell disease in a patient from a susceptible racial group.

176   Fanconi's anaemia. ▶
This is a rare form of anaemia, the features of which include hypoplasia of the thumbs, radii and first metacarpals. In this example, the thumbs (A) and particularly the right first metacarpal (B) are hypoplastic.

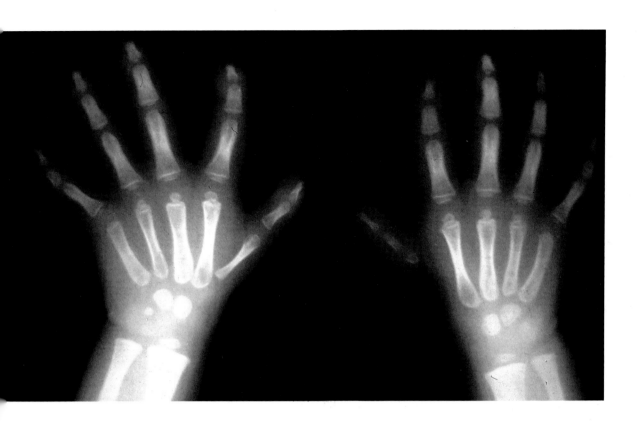

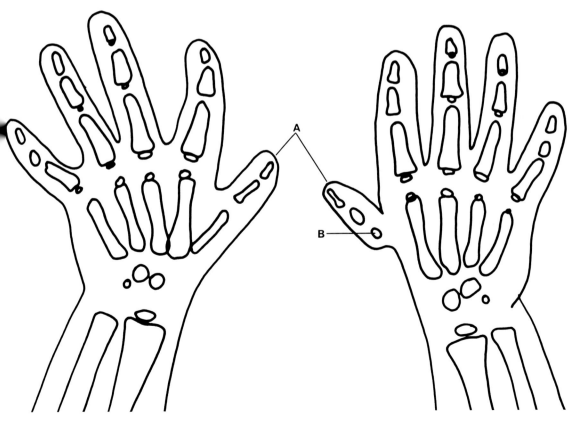

209

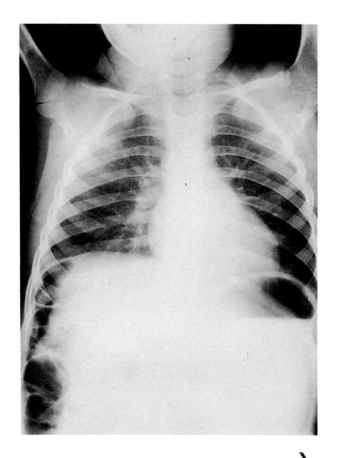

177   Leukaemia.
Leukaemic changes in bone are due to
leukaemic infiltration of the marrow. The
type of leukaemia cannot be inferred from
the radiological changes. Horizontal lucent
bands in the metaphyses are common and,
in this example, are shown in the humeral
necks (A). There is also periosteal reaction
(B) along the humeral shafts.

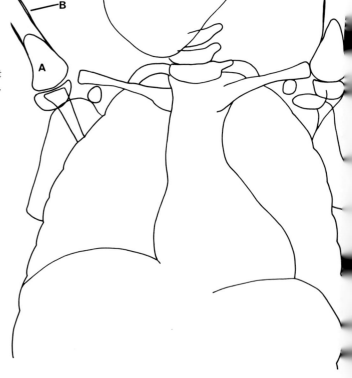

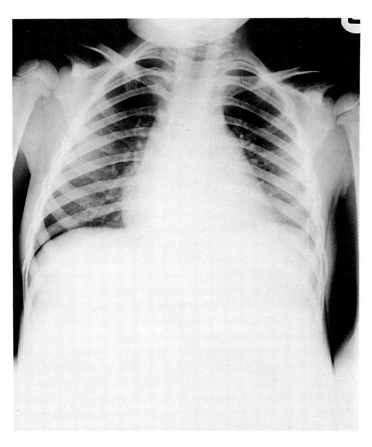

178 Acute lymphocytic leukaemia.
Sometimes the banding is not seen and
only subtle cortical metaphyseal erosions
(A) are present, as in this case, involving
the proximal humeri.

211

179 **Chronic myeloid leukaemia.**
In adults, usually only in chronic leukaemia is there time for bony changes to develop. Bone changes are more common in children.

(a) *PA view of chest.*
In this example, there is irregular destruction of the humerus (A) with some sclerosis (B). There is an associated soft tissue mass with disorganised new bone formation (C). Several of the other bones of the thoracic cage and upper limb girdle have a rather 'moth-eaten' appearance and are probably involved. There is bilateral pleural thickening due to the presence of leukaemic deposits (D). The superior mediastinum is widened secondary to lymph node enlargement (E). These changes cannot be differentiated from carcinomatosis on radiological grounds alone.

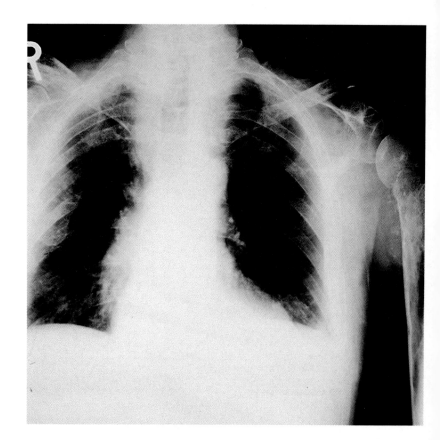

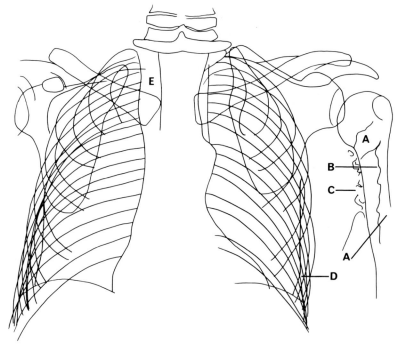

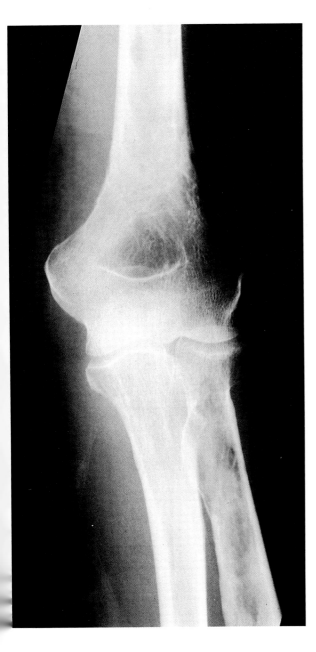
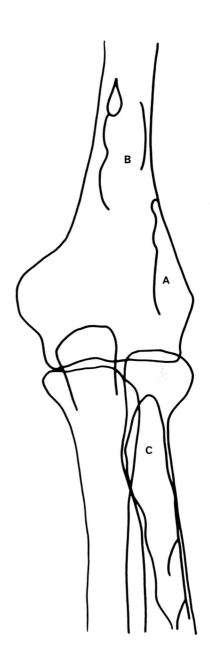

(b)   *Elbow of the same patient.*
There is loss of bone density over the lateral aspect of the distal humerus (A) and a scalloped, lucent medullary pattern in the distal humerus (B). The proximal radius has a similar appearance and shows endosteal bony expansion (C).

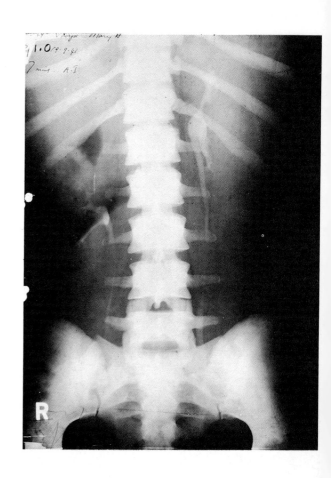

180 Myelofibrosis.
There is replacement of the marrow by
fibrous tissue, giving rise to a sclerotic
appearance. It may end in leukaemia and so
is one of a spectrum of myeloproliferative
disorders.
The radiological sign most usually seen is of
increased bone density, in this case in the
ribs, thoracic spine, lumbo-sacral spine and
pelvis.
In some cases, the increased density and
obliteration of the marrow cavity are
sufficiently severe to resemble
osteopetrosis, fluorosis or widespread
osteoblastic metastases.

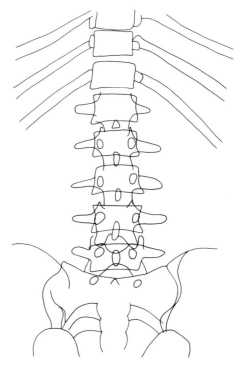

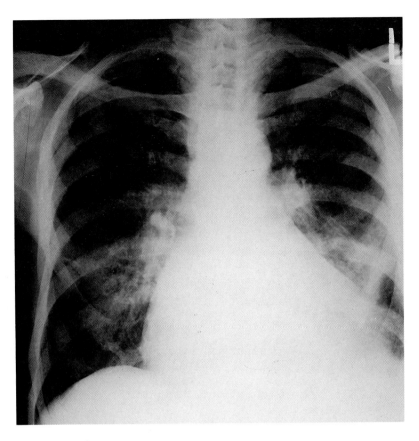

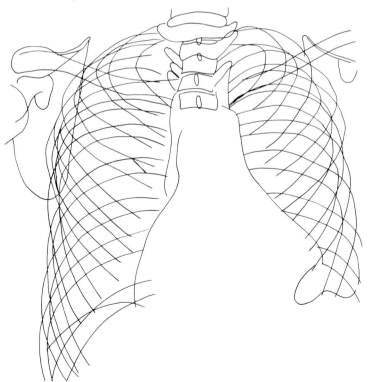

181   Myelofibrosis—chest. There is increased bone density with some bony expansion in the upper limb girdle and thoracic cage. The condition may be recognised first on a chest x-ray, as such an examination is performed so frequently, often for non-specific reasons.

215

8: ENDOCRINE AND METABOLIC BONE DISEASE

Bone growth, development and mineralisation are involved in several metabolic pathways, some of which are under endocrine control. Endocrine and metabolic disease is, therefore, often manifested in the skeleton.

Disorders of bone density, mineralisation, growth and maturation occur. Weakened bone is prone to pathological fracture.

Many of these abnormalities, singly or in combination, are shown in the following illustrations.

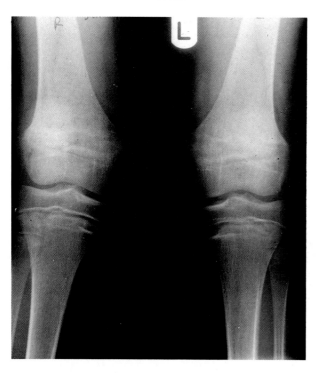

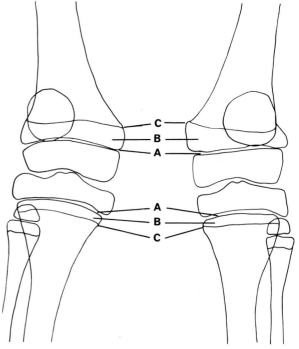

182   **Rickets.**
Classical dietary rickets is due to dietary lack of calcium and vitamin D. Typical dietary rickets is relatively rare in Western children.
The radiological changes are due to deficient mineralisation of osteoid in growing children and are hence most marked in the metaphyses.

(a)   AP view of knees.
The first case is one of recurrent rickets following partial treatment. The epiphyseal plates (A) are relatively wide and there are broad, distal metaphyseal lucent bands (B). Immediately under the bands, there are transverse sclerotic lines (C) indicating that the process has been arrested and has re-started. This is a sign of partial or intermittent treatment. Similar changes are seen in the ankles and wrists.

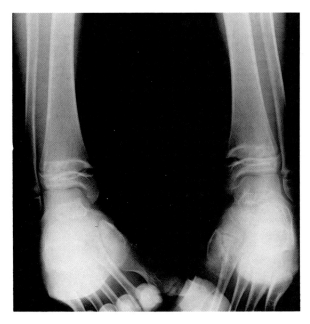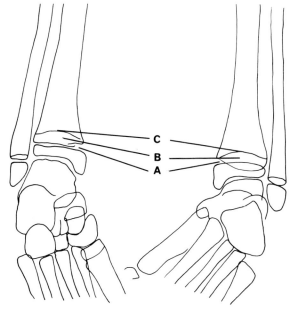

(b) The ankles.

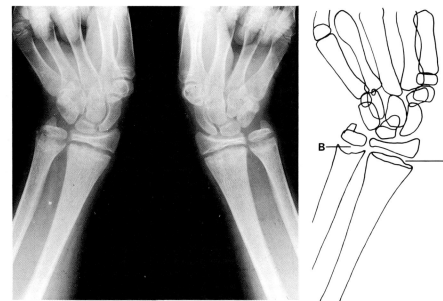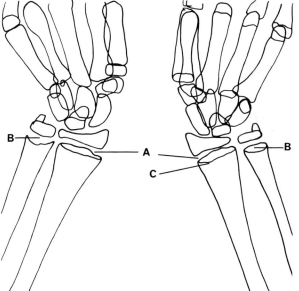

(c) The wrists.

217

183   Hypophosphataemic rickets.

In this familial condition, there is renal loss of phosphate. The radiological appearance is the same as in dietary rickets but the patient does not respond to normal doses of vitamin D.

(a)   Hands.

There are marked rachitic changes in the wrist and hand of this African child who presented with severe rickets and did not respond to vitamin D.
(A) There are wide, lucent, metaphyseal bands merging with the widened epiphyseal plates.
(B) The metaphyseal edges have a frayed or 'rotting-stump' appearance.
(C) There is abnormal bone modelling peripherally.
(D) The margins of several of the phalanges are irregular due to subperiosteal bone resorption. Both this and the 'rotting-stump' appearance occur in secondary hyperparathyroidism which is present in this case.

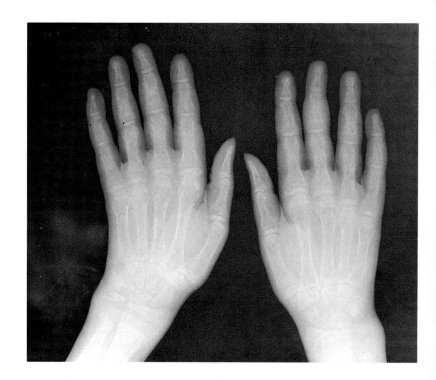

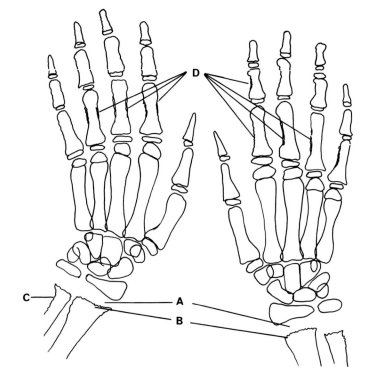

218

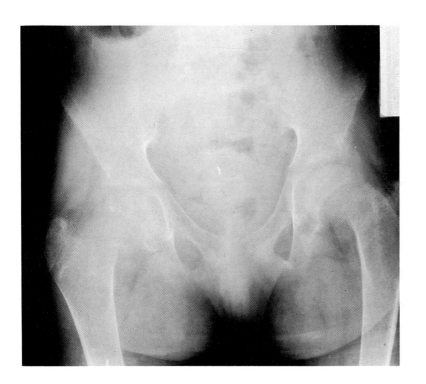

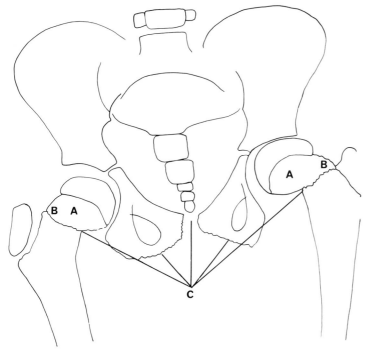

(b) *The pelvis and hips of the same patient.*
Severe changes are also shown in the pelvis and hips.
(A) There are wide femoral metaphyseal bands.
(B) The femoral necks are bowed with bilateral varus deformities.
(C) The femoral metaphyses, the pubic symphysis and the inferior margins of the pubic bones have a 'frayed' appearance.

219

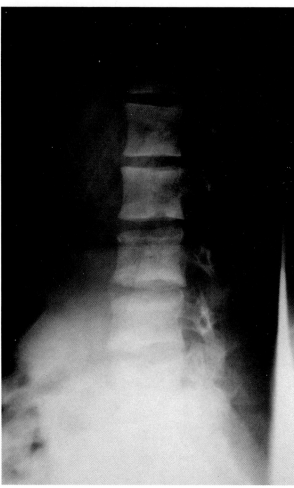

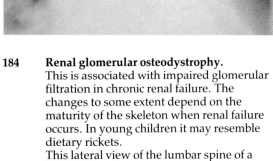

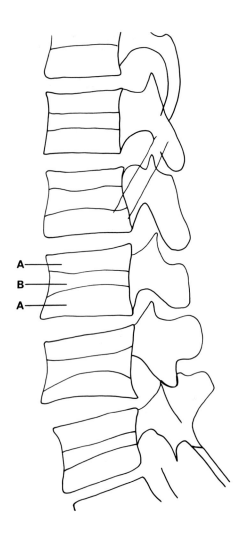

184   **Renal glomerular osteodystrophy.**
This is associated with impaired glomerular
filtration in chronic renal failure. The
changes to some extent depend on the
maturity of the skeleton when renal failure
occurs. In young children it may resemble
dietary rickets.
This lateral view of the lumbar spine of a

young adult exhibits the 'rugger-jersey'
appearance which is characteristic of the
condition but is not exclusive to it. There is
increased bone density (A) over the disc
margins, with a relative decrease in density
(B) in the centre of the vertebral body.

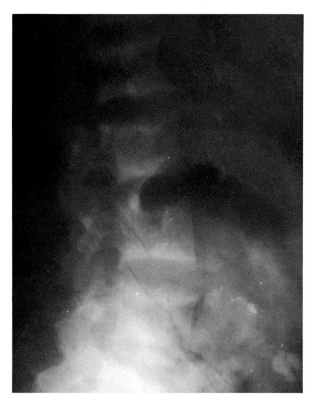

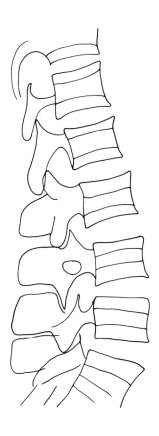

185   Primary hyperparathyroidism.

(a) *Lateral lumbar spine.*
This is another example of a 'rugger-jersey' spine, showing that it is not exclusive to renal glomerular osteodystrophy. The changes in the latter are due to secondary hyperparathyroidism.

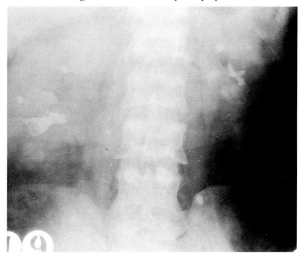

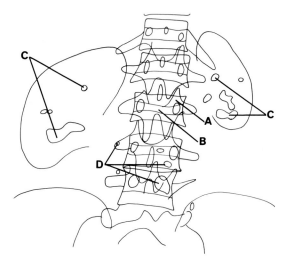

(b) *The AP view of the abdomen of the same patient.*
The alternating sclerotic (A) and lucent bands (B) of the 'rugger-jersey' spine are seen again. Bilateral renal calculi (C) are present. These may be the first evidence of hyperparathyroidism. There are also calcified mesenteric lymph nodes (D) but these are common in normal individuals.

221

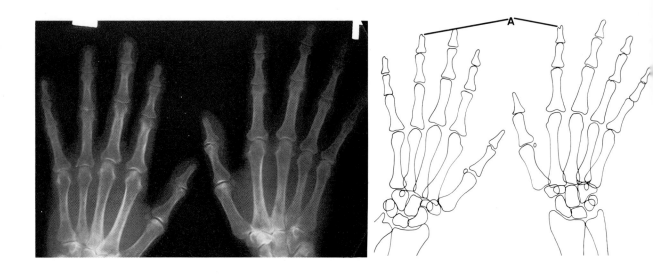

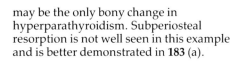

(c) *The hands of the same patient.*
There is erosion of the terminal tufts of several distal phalanges (A). This finding, along with subperiosteal resorption of the phalangeal shafts, is usually the first, and may be the only bony change in hyperparathyroidism. Subperiosteal resorption is not well seen in this example and is better demonstrated in **183** (a).

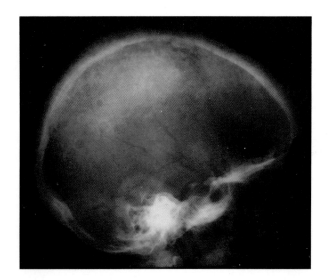

(d) *Skull—same patient.*
There are multiple tiny lucencies (A) in the skull vault, the so-called 'pepper-pot' skull.

222

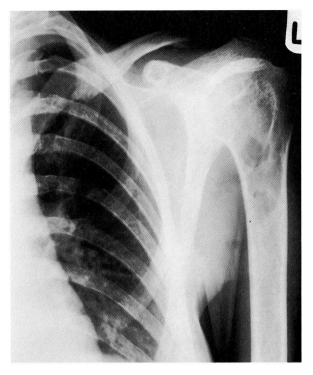
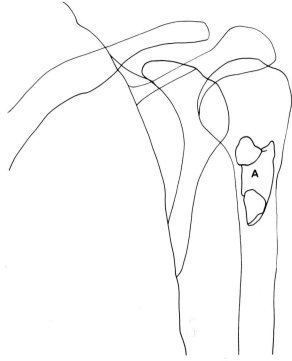

186 **Primary hyperparathyroidism.**
Brown tumour of upper humerus. There is
a well-defined, partly loculated, lucent
defect (A) in the upper humerus.
In the absence of other evidence of
hyperparathyroidism, or when a single

bone is viewed in isolation, it is easy to
forget hyperparathyroidism in the
differential diagnosis of bone cysts and
tumours.

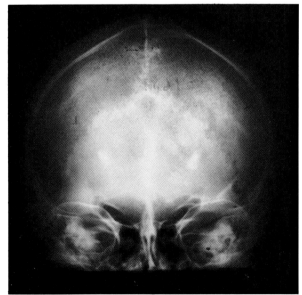
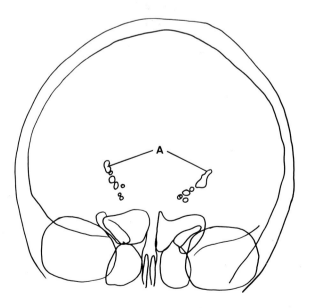

187 **Hypoparathyroidism.**
The main radiological feature is ectopic
calcification, most often seen in the basal
ganglia of the brain (A).

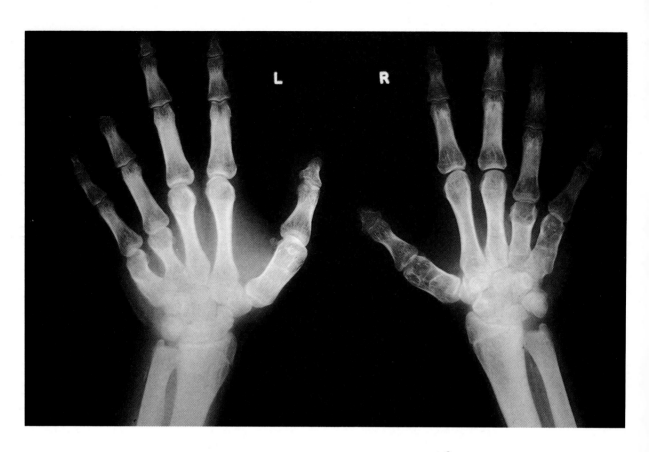

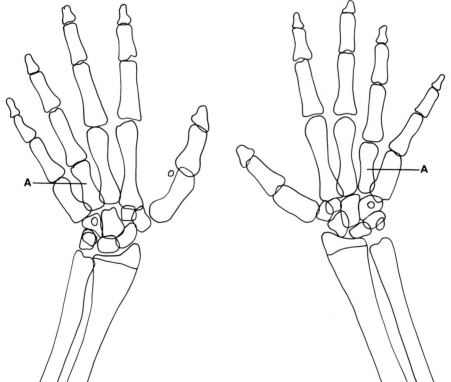

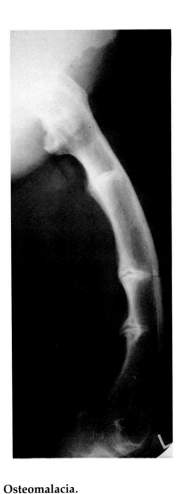

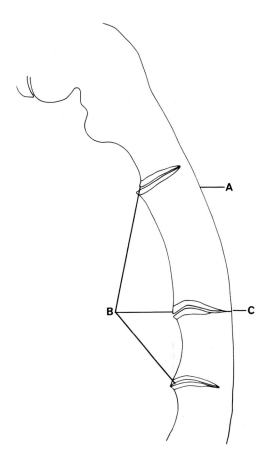

189　**Osteomalacia.**
When an adult is deprived of calcium or vitamin D, osteomalacia occurs rather than rickets. The bones show demineralisation and deformity secondary to softening. This example, in the femur, shows marked anterior bowing (A) and Looser's zones (B). These Looser's zones are due to defective healing of stress fractures by osteoid rather than new bone. Osteoid causes the dense margins of the stress fracture lines. Looser's zones are characteristic of osteomalacia. One of them has extended across the femoral shaft to cause a complete fracture (C).

188　**Pseudohypoparathyroidism.**
◄　This is a rare condition, of autosomal dominant inheritance. The biochemical changes are similar to those of hypoparathyroidism but there is no response to parathormone.
Radiological changes include basal ganglia calcification, as in true hypoparathyroidism. Short stature, particularly with short fourth and fifth metacarpals (A) is the salient radiological feature.

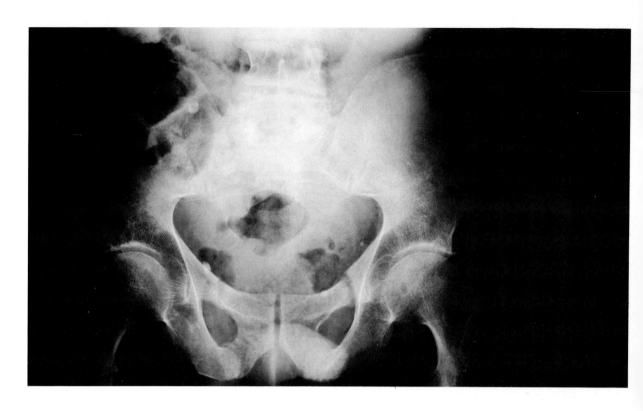

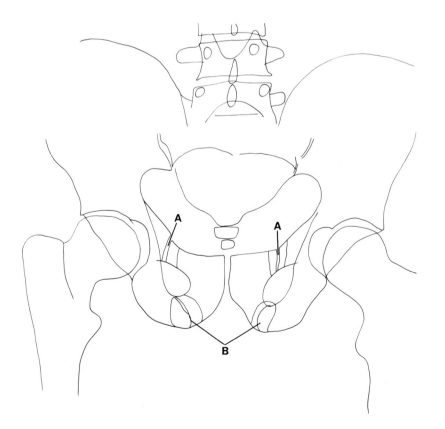

190 Osteomalacia of the pelvis. There are Looser's zones in the superior (A) and inferior pubic rami (B), characteristic sites.

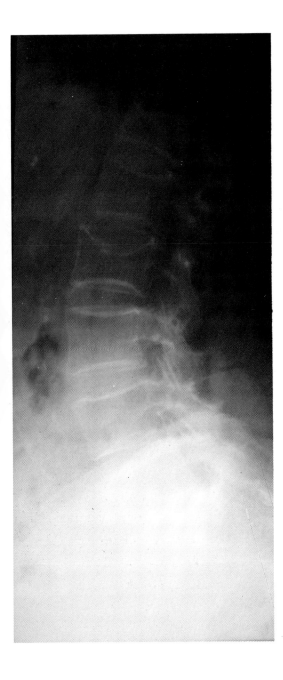
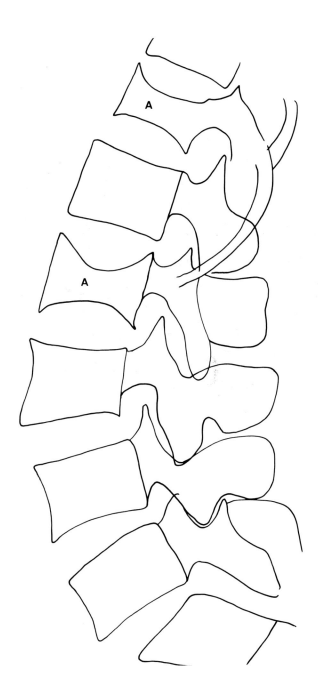

191   Osteoporosis.
Whereas osteomalacia is due to deficient mineralisation of osteoid, osteoporosis is due to deficient bone formation. In the early stages, loss of bone density is common to both disorders and differentiation may be difficult. Osteoporosis is much more common than osteomalacia and is present to some extent in most of the ageing population, particularly female. It is also caused, by steroid therapy.

Osteomalacic bone tends to bend but osteoporotic bone breaks readily and fractures, particularly of the femoral necks and vertebral bodies, are common.

This lateral view of the lumbar spine shows loss of bone density and partial loss of height of two vertebrae (A), due to compression fractures.

192 Hypothyroidism— cretinism.
Skeletal growth and maturation depend on thyroid hormone among other factors. If thyroid hormone is lacking from birth, cretinism is the result. Fortunately, it is rarely seen nowadays. The examples shown are of an untreated patient who presented in adult life.

(a) *Skull.*
The bones of the vault (A) and base (B) are thickened. The sutures are prominent and a few sutural (Wormian) bones can be seen (C).

(b) *Lateral thoracic and lumbar spine showing gross platyspondyly.*
All of the vertebrae are flattened and some of the apophyses (A) have not fused. The sacral segments (B) are still separate.
These changes and the changes in the epiphyses resemble certain of the the mucopolysaccharidoses. This patient was originally thought to be a gargoyle (MPS I) and thyroid treatment was not given. Hence the full-blown appearance in adult life.

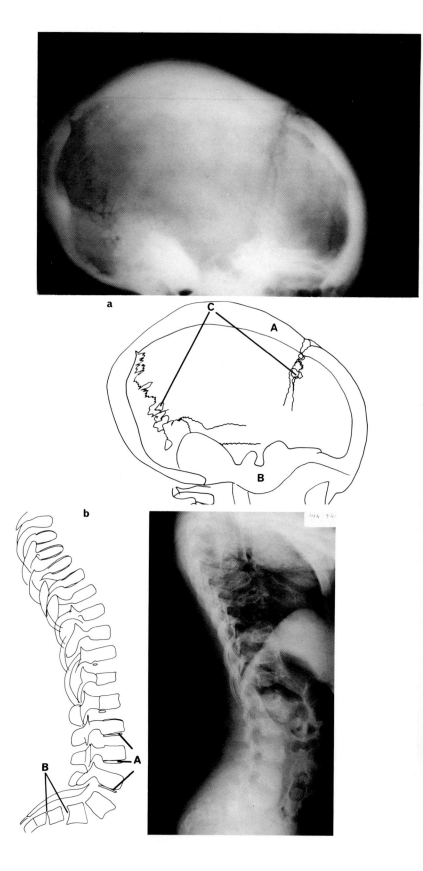

228

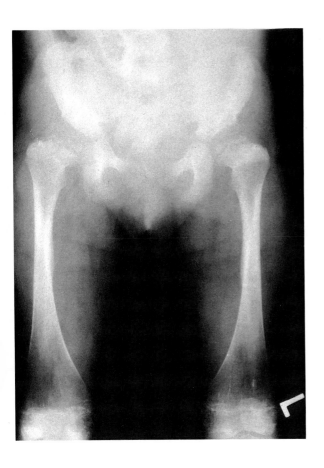
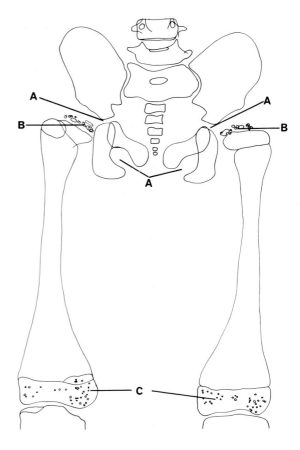

(c) *Immature appearance of the
     pelvis.*
     (A) The pelvic bones are
     unfused with wide
     synchondroses.
     (B) The proximal
     femoral epiphyses are
     unfused, flattened and
     stippled.
     (C) The distal femoral
     epiphyses have more
     normal shape but are
     still unfused and
     stippled.

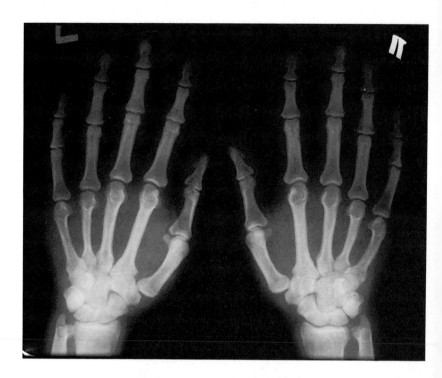

193 Acromegaly.
Acromegaly is caused by the production of excess growth hormone from an eosinophilic adenoma or hyperplasia of the pituitary gland. In a child, excess growth hormone leads to gigantism.

(a) *Hands.*
The hands are large, with expanded, spade-like, terminal phalangeal tufts (A).

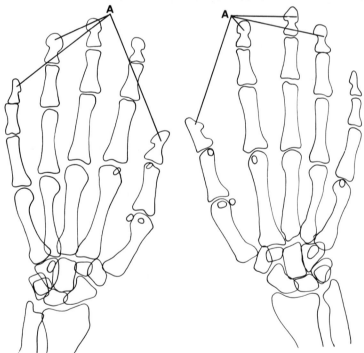

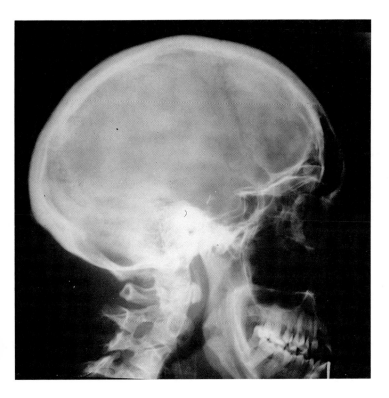

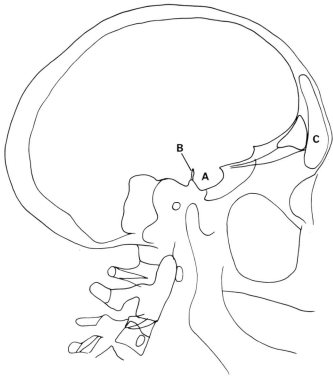

(b)   *Lateral skull.*
The sella (A) is enlarged and its dorsum (B) is eroded due to expansion from within by a eosinophil adenoma.
The frontal sinuses (C) are large but within normal limits in this case.

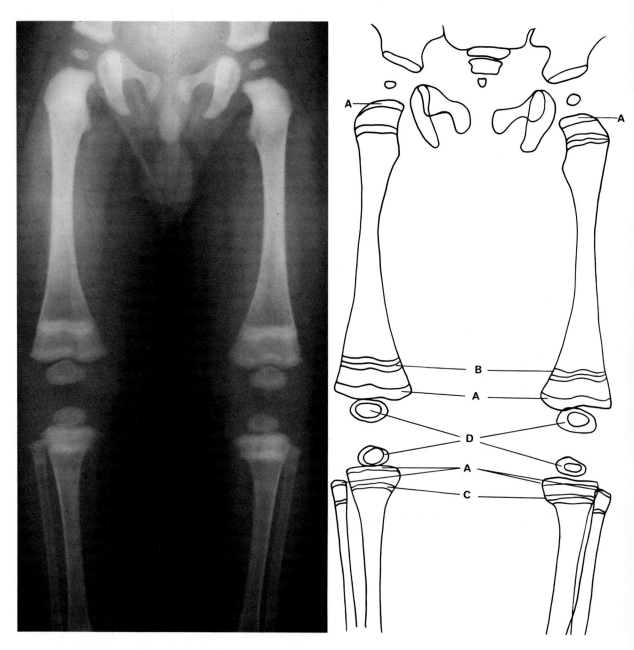

194   Lead poisoning.
Lead deposition in growing bone causes a
dense metaphyseal band (A). In this case,
the presence of further submetaphyseal
bands, particularly in the distal femora (B)
and proximal tibiae (C), indicated that the
poisoning was intermittent. The presence
of dense circles (D) within the epiphyses
has the same meaning.

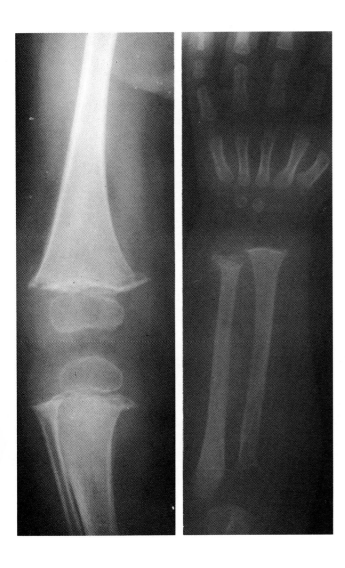

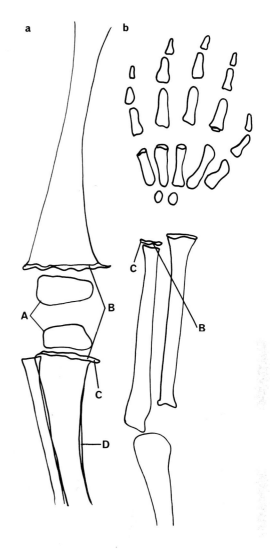

195 **Scurvy.**
This is rarely seen in developed countries. Lack of vitamin C leads to deficient formation of osteoid and hence osteoporosis.

(a) Right knee.
In this example, there is osteoporosis with a thin rim of increased density around the distal femoral and proximal tibial epiphyses (A). Sub-metaphyseal fractures (B) lead to the beak-like 'Pelkan's spur' (C). Sub-periosteal haematoma and subsequent calcification becomes visible along bone shafts (D).

(b) Forearm, wrist and hand.
This picture shows osteoporosis, an ulnar submetaphyseal fracture (B) and Pelkan's spur (C).

233

9: CONGENITAL ABNORMALITIES

Most students find the radiological diagnosis of congenital abnormalities a difficult subject. However, the more common abnormalities should be recognised relatively easily.

Many abnormalities are isolated, affecting single bones and are of no other significance. Some isolated bony anomalies may be associated with congenital abnormalities in other systems.

When several bones are abnormal, particularly when a disorder of growth is present, it is important to look at the sites and distribution of radiological changes. It is useful to know whether the axial or peripheral skeleton is more involved, whether the proximal or distal limb bones are more affected and whether the epiphyses, metaphyses or diaphyses of long bones are involved. For instance, it is essential to know that in achondroplasia bone shortening affects the proximal, more than the distal, limb bones.

It is also important to note if the bone texture is primarily sclerotic as in osteopetrosis or osteopaenic as in osteogenesis imperfecta.

More specific findings will be mentioned subsequently in the text.

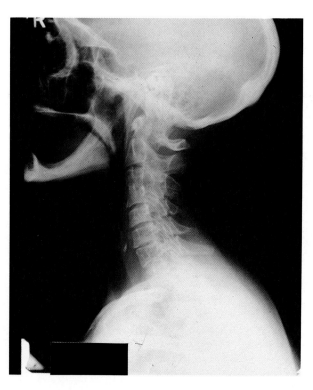
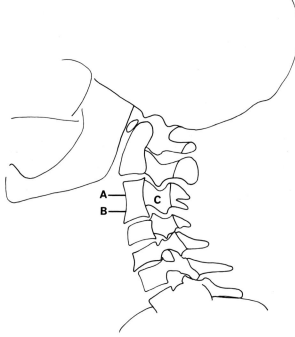

196   **Block vertebrae.**

(a) *Lateral view.*
There is congenital fusion of the third (A) and fourth (B) cervical vertebral bodies and their neural arches (C). The bodies are narrowed in AP diameter. These features help distinguish this congenital disorder from an acquired post-inflammatory fusion of the vertebral bodies, in which the arches usually remain separate. An exception is juvenile rheumatoid arthritis in which the arches may fuse.
A more severe version of this anomaly is the Klippel-Feil syndrome in which several adjacent vertebrae are fused, the neck is short and there are often other associated congenital abnormalities.

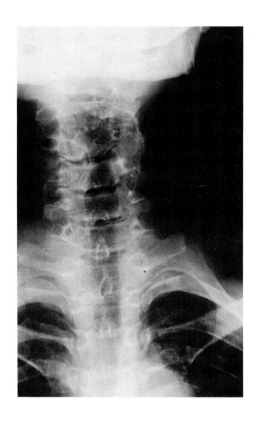
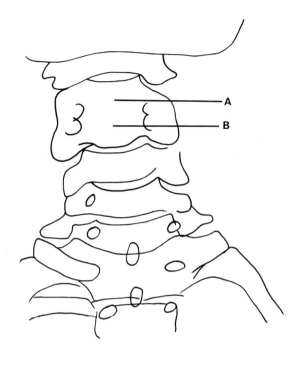

(b) *AP view.*
The fusion of the vertebral bodies (A and B) is less clearly seen than on the lateral view.

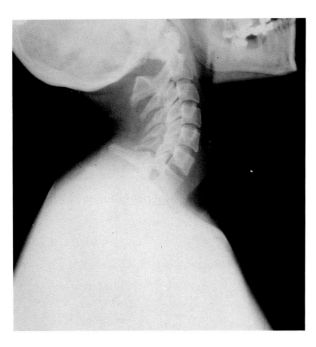

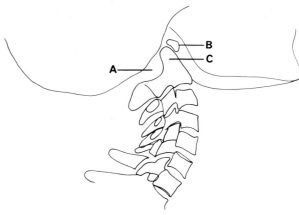

197 **Congenital absence of posterior arch of atlas.**

(a) *Lateral view in extension.*
The posterior arch of the atlas is absent (A).
The gap between the anterior arch of the
atlas (B) and the odontoid peg of the axis
(C) is normal.

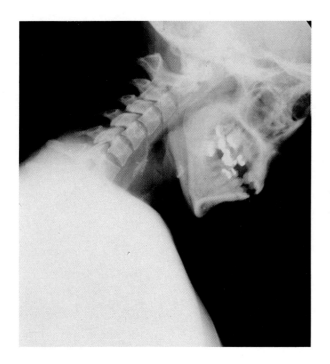

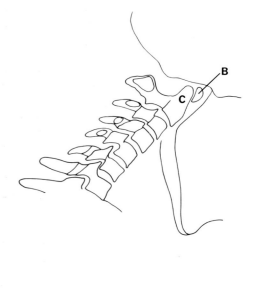

(b) *The same patient—lateral view in flexion.*
The gap between the anterior arch of the
atlas (B) and the odontoid (C) has not
increased. The joint is, therefore, stable.

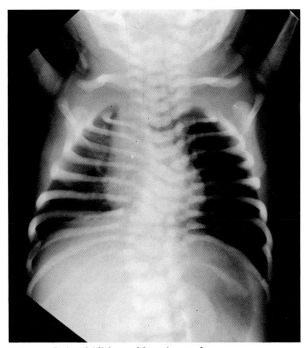

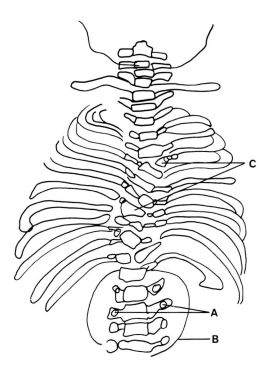

198 Spina bifida and hemi-vertebrae.

(a)   AP view.
The interpedicular distances in the lumbar spine are widened (A). The soft tissue shadow of the associated meningocele can be seen (B). There are also several hemi-vertebrae (C) in the mid and lower thoracic spine with associated scoliosis. Combinations of vertebral anomalies like this are common.

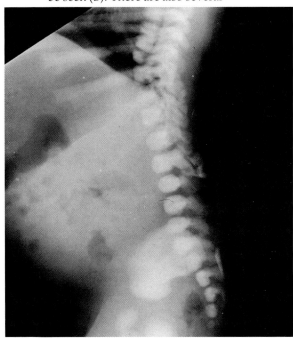

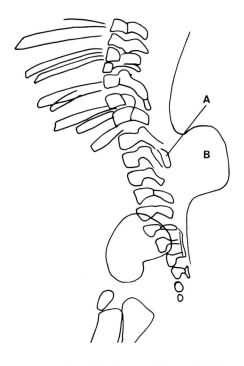

(b)   The same patient—lateral view.
The bony defects are not so well seen but the arch of the second lumbar vertebra (A) is abnormal and the faint soft tissue shadow of the meningocele projects posteriorly (B).

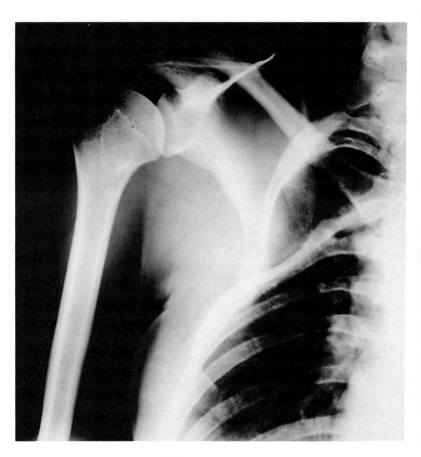

199 Sprengel's shoulder.
The scapula is high and
malrotated with shortening
of its vertebral border (A).
The malrotation is causing
the scapula to impinge on
and deform the third rib
(B). The scapula may be
attached to the cervical
spine by the omo-vertebral
bone (not seen in this case).
Other anomalies such as
hemi-vertebrae and the
Klippel-Feil syndrome may
be associated.

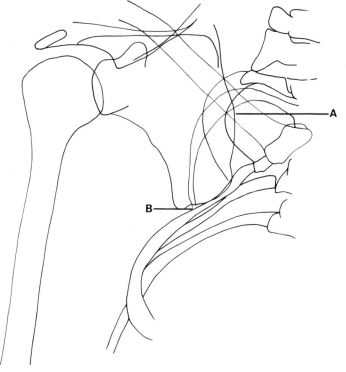

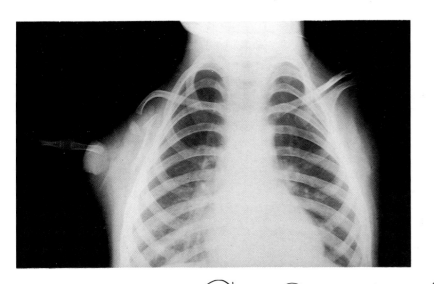

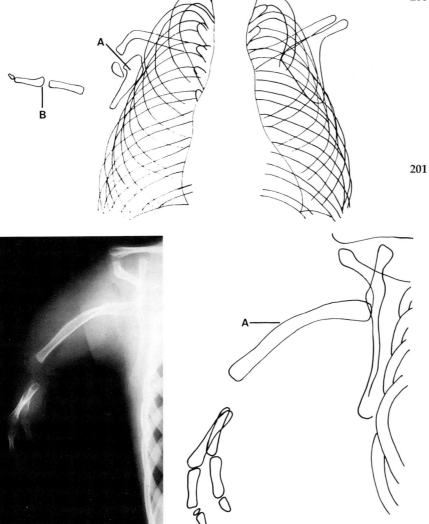

200 **Phocomelia of the upper limb.**
The proximal limb bones are absent. In this case, only the remnants of the scapula (A) and right thumb (B) can be seen, the thumb arising from the shoulder. This is the characteristic deformity caused by thalidomide.

201 **Phocomelia.**
Another case, showing absence of the humerus and a single deformed distal forearm bone (A).

239

202 Hemimelia.
Absence of the distal limb
bones. Distal to the elbow,
only the olecranon (A) and
the radial head (B) are
present. The bone distal to
these remnants is absent.

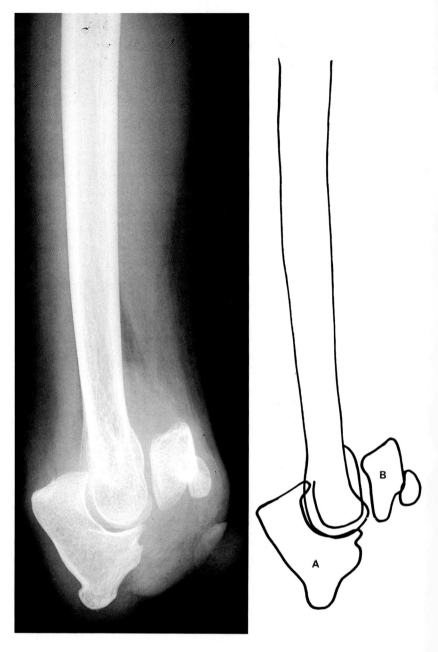

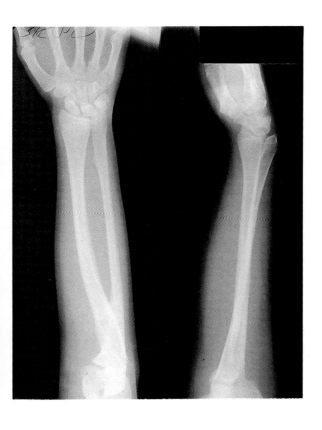

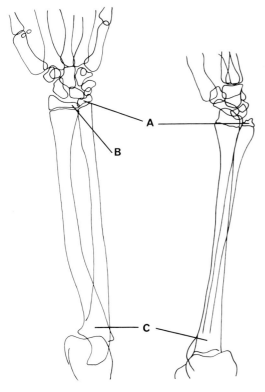

203 Madelung's deformity.
The ulna is bowed posteriorly and its distal end
(A) is projected behind the wrist. This anomaly
is considered to be secondary to shortening of
the radius and hypoplasia of the ulnar aspect of
the distal radial epiphysis (B). It is usually
bilateral. In this example, there is also fusion of
the proximal ends of the radius and ulna (C).

241

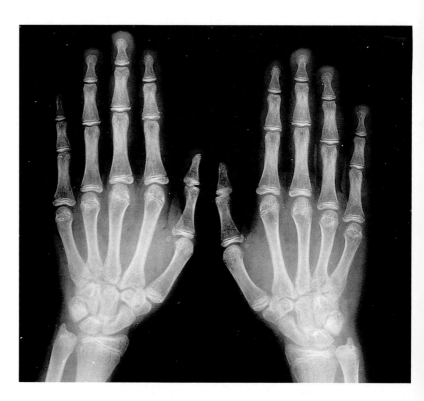

204 Turner's syndrome.
The fourth metacarpals (A)
are a little shortened. The
shortening is not
particularly marked in this
example. Other skeletal
abnormalities may be seen,
including deformities of the
hands, feet, knees and
cervical spine. There may
be retarded bone
maturation but final adult
stature is usually short.

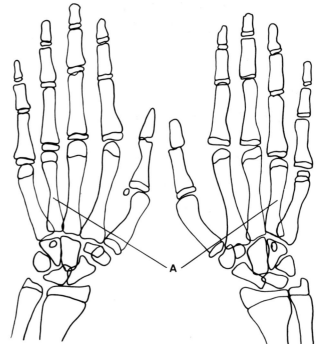

242

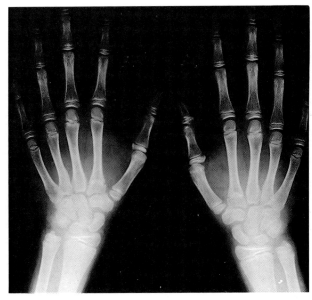
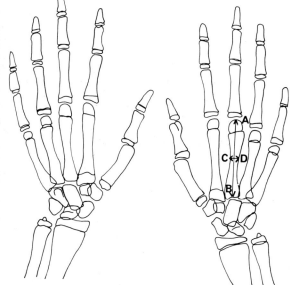

205   Marfan's syndrome.

(a) *Hands.*

The fingers are long and slender. Arachnodactyly is assessed by measuring the lengths (A-B) of the 2nd, 3rd, 4th and 5th metacarpals and dividing them by their widths (C-D) at the exact mid-points. The total of the four lengths divided by the total of the four widths gives the metacarpal index. The normal range is 5.4 to 7.9. This range does not apply to individuals of African origin in whom the upper limit of normal is up to 9 in males and 9.5 in females. In this case, the metacarpal index is 9.7, well above the upper limit of normal. The patient was considered to have Marfan's syndrome although this cannot be diagnosed on metacarpal index alone.

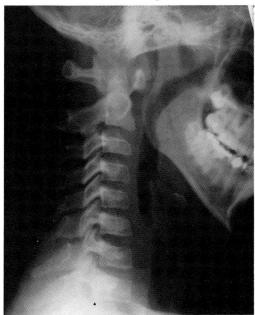
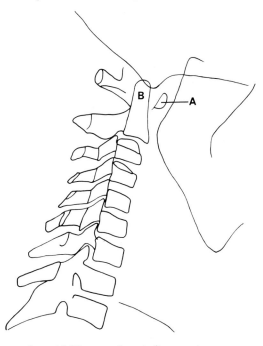

(b) *The same patient—view of the lateral cervical spine.*

There is an increase in joint width between the anterior arch of the atlas (A) and the odontoid (B) secondary to ligamentous laxity.

243

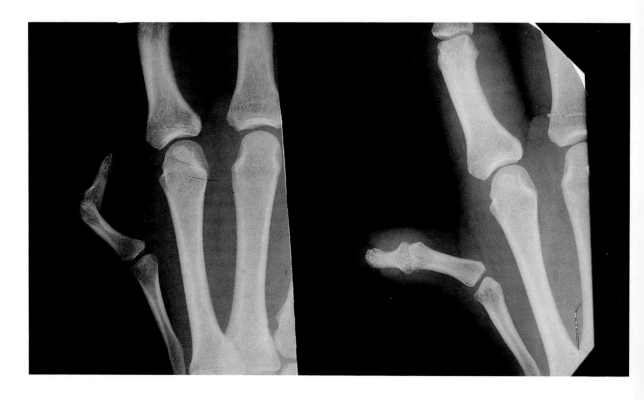

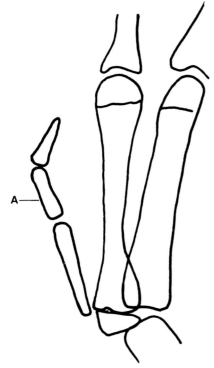

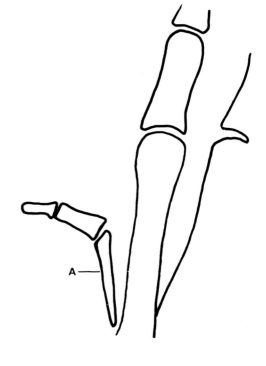

206 **Hypoplasia of thumb.**
There is a small, hypoplastic thumb (A).
Such hypoplasia may occur in association
with other conditions such as Fanconi's
anaemia and Holt-Oram syndrome. In this
case, it is an isolated anomaly.

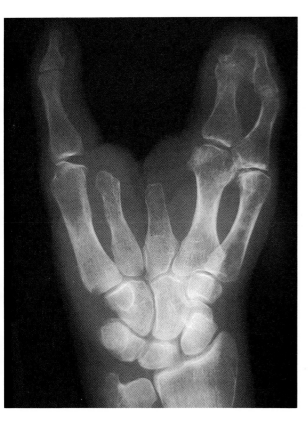

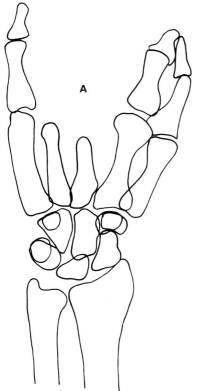

207   **Lobster-claw hand.**
The phalanges of the third and fourth digits are absent, causing a deep cleft (A) in the hand.

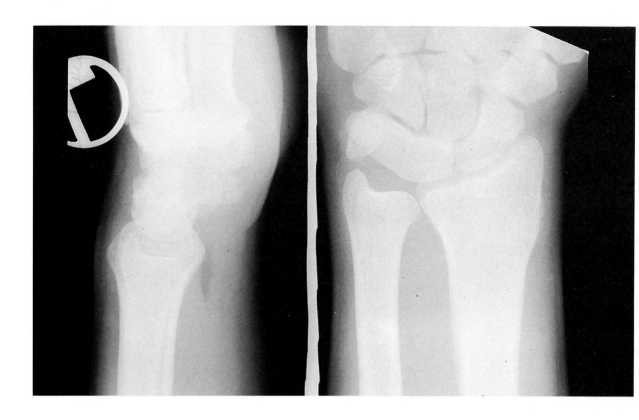

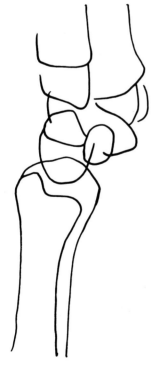

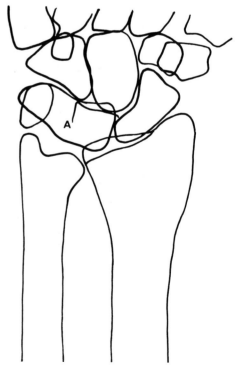

208   Congenital carpal fusion.
There is fusion of the lunate and triquetral (A). As with other hand abnormalities, fusion may occur as part of a syndrome or may be an isolated anomaly, as in this case.

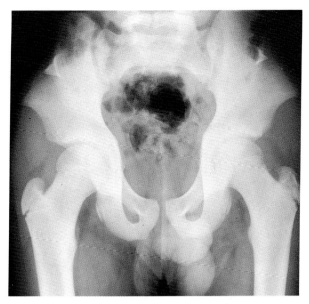

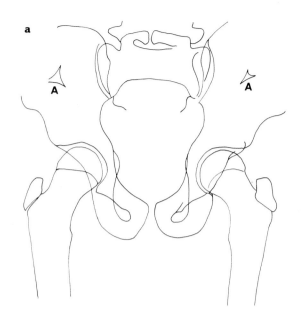

209   Fong's syndrome—nail-patella syndrome.

(a) *AP view of pelvis.*
This syndrome includes a combination of
hypoplastic nails, iliac horns and absent or
hypoplastic patellae. Bilateral bony horns
(A) are seen projecting posteriorly from the
ilia.

(b) *Fong's syndrome.*
The same patient has hypoplastic patellae.
One is shown (A).

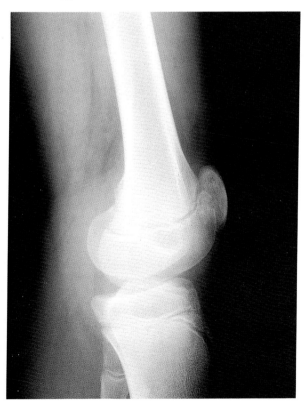

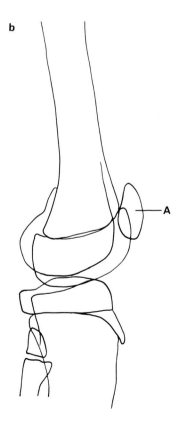

210 Bilateral congenital dislocation of the hips.
The femoral heads are not ossified but the femoral necks (A) can be seen displaced laterally from the shallow acetabula (B). This is obvious dislocation and lesser degrees may be missed radiologically. The pelvis is best x-rayed, not in the neutral position, but with straight legs abducted 45 degrees and internally rotated (diagram). A line drawn through the femoral shaft usually crosses the lumbo-sacral joint (C) in the normal infant. If the joint is dislocated, this line (L) will pass through the ipsi-lateral ilium (D).

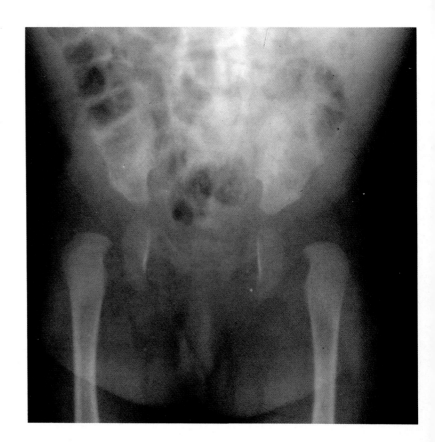

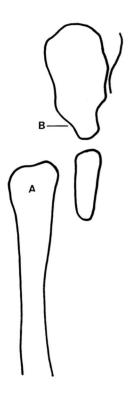

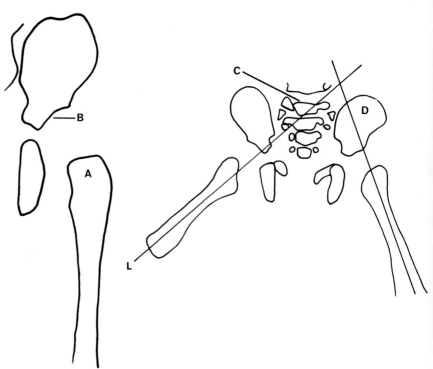

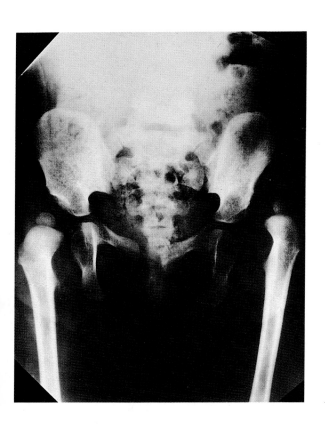

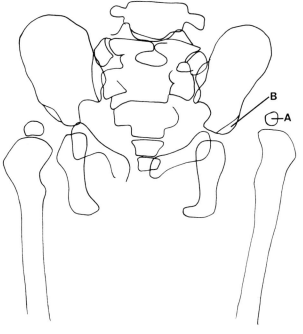

211 **Congenital dislocation of the left hip.**
The left femoral head (A) is smaller than the
right as a result of delayed ossification. It is
completely displaced from the shallow
acetabulum (B).

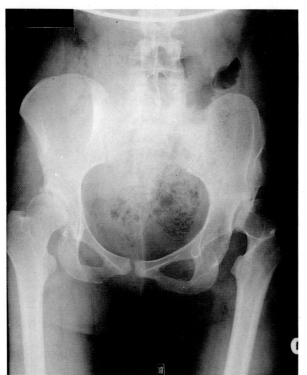
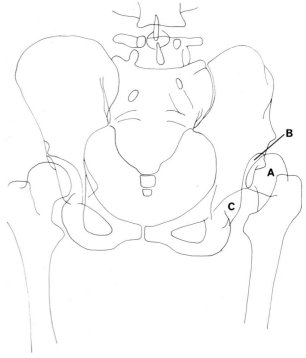

212 **Congenital dislocation of the left hip—late deformity.**
The femoral head (A) is flattened and is situated in a false acetabulum (B). Without the femoral head in place, the true acetabulum (C) has failed to develop normally.

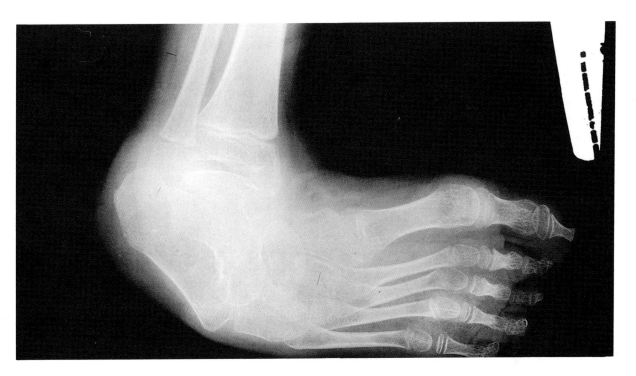

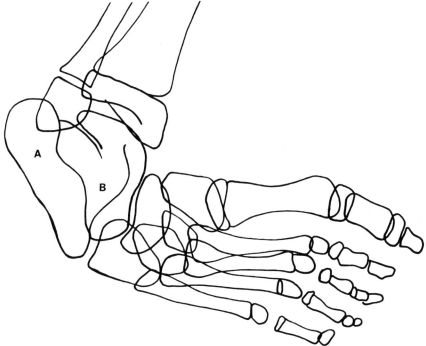

213   Club-foot—talipes equinovarus.
This relatively common abnormality is easily recognised clinically. There is some debate as to whether radiology adds much to the diagnosis or management. It is usually an isolated anomaly but may be unilateral or bilateral. It may also occur in other conditions such as neurological abnormalities and arthrogryposis multiplex congenita. This film shows the uncorrected abnormality in an older child. The calcaneus (A) is malrotated and the talus (B) has taken up a more vertical position than usual.

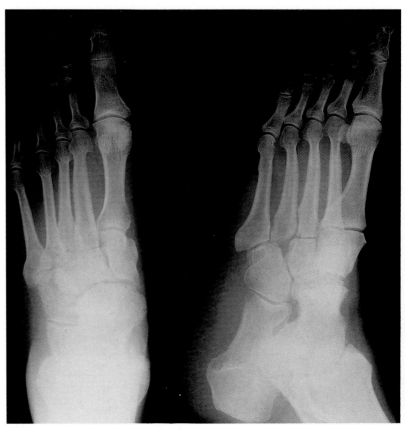

214 **Talo-navicular fusion.**
There is a bar of bone (A)
joining the talus and
navicular in the oblique
view. There is associated
osteoarthritis of the distal
articular surface of the
navicular with osteophyte
formation (B).
Talo-calcaneal and
calcaneo-navicular fusions
are common and may lead
to the spastic type of flat
foot which presents in adult
life. The common simple
flat foot is not associated
with tarsal fusions.

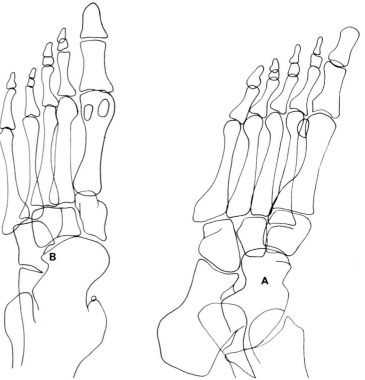

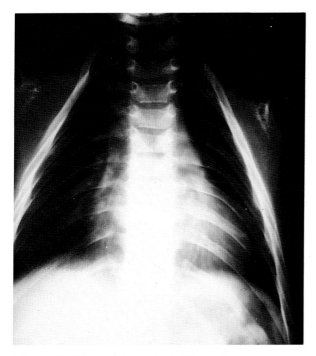
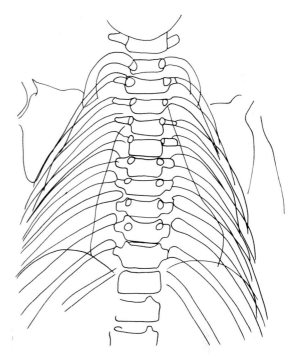

215 **Cleidocranial dysplasia (formerly dysostosis).**

(a) AP view of chest.
There is defective ossification of bone, leading to absence of the outer ends or all of the clavicles, Wormian bones in the skull and pelvic deformities including coxa vara. This film shows absence of the clavicles.

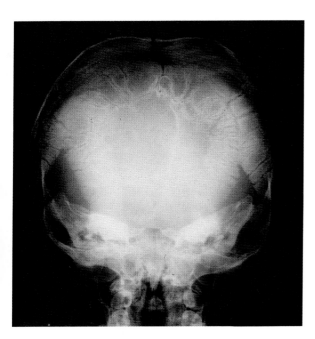
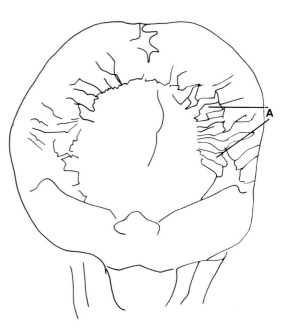

(b) Cleidocranial dysplasia.
The skull sutures have excessive interdigitations and contain multiple Wormian (sutural) bones (A).

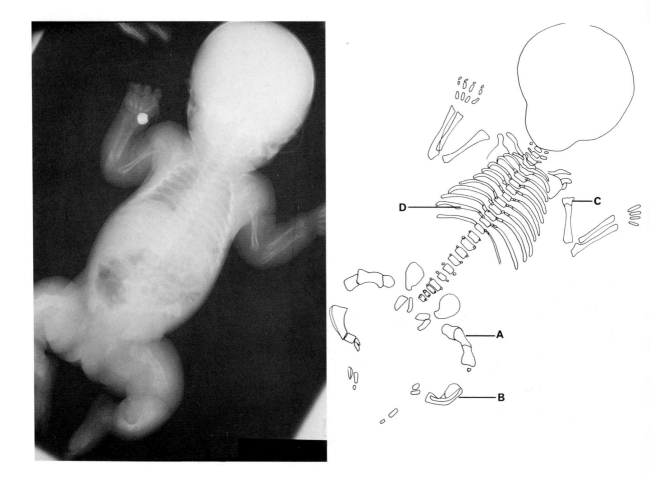

216   Osteogenesis imperfecta.
This condition is a result of inadequate osteogenesis and leads to multiple fractures. These heal, often with abundant callus, and secondary deformities are common. Infantile, intermediate and adult types are described in decreasing order of frequency.

This example shows multiple fractures in various stages of healing and secondary deformities in the infantile type. The fractures and deformities are most marked in the femora (A) and tibiae (B). There are also fractures of the left proximal humeral metaphysis (C) and at least one rib (D).

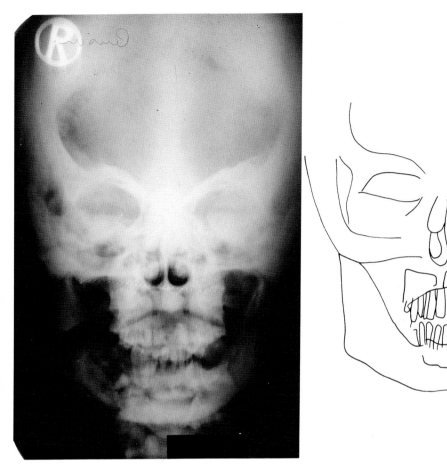

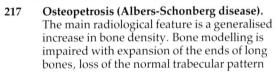

217 Osteopetrosis (Albers-Schonberg disease).
The main radiological feature is a generalised
increase in bone density. Bone modelling is
impaired with expansion of the ends of long
bones, loss of the normal trabecular pattern

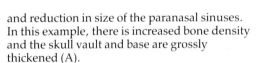

and reduction in size of the paranasal sinuses.
In this example, there is increased bone density
and the skull vault and base are grossly
thickened (A).

218   Melorrheostosis.

(a) *AP view of tibia.*

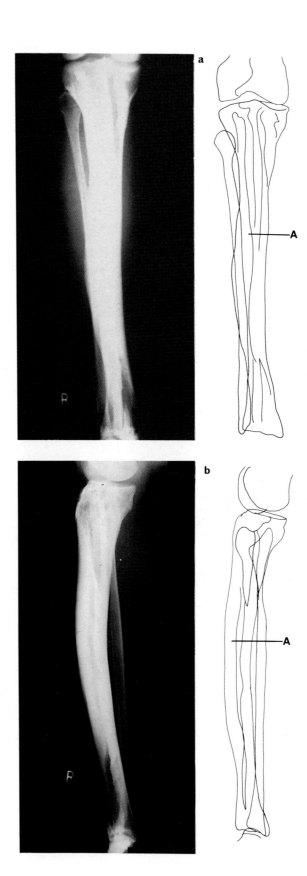

(b) *Lateral view of tibia.*
This is a rare condition of unknown aetiology. It may involve one or several bones and, apart from local deformity, is generally of little significance. The pattern of hyperostosis has been likened to wax flowing down a candle. This type of eccentric sclerosis (A) is shown in a tibia.

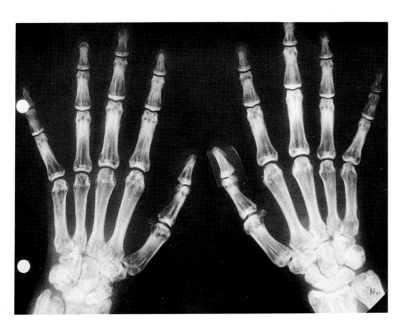

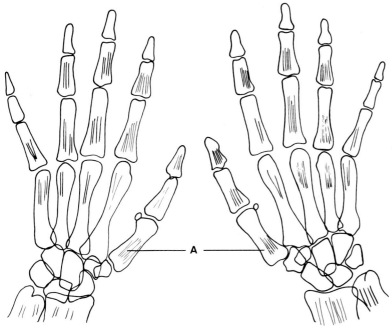

219   Osteopathia striata.
This is a radiological
curiosity of no clinical
importance.
Dense striations (A) are
seen running longitudinally
in long bones, in this case in
the hands.

257

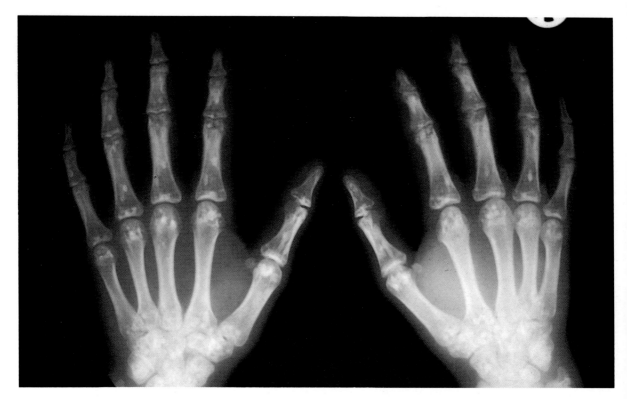

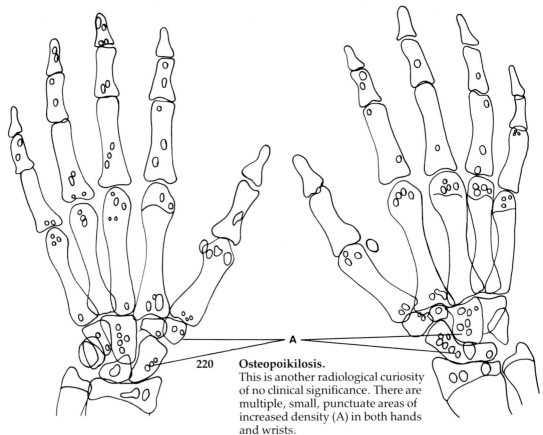

A

220 Osteopoikilosis.
This is another radiological curiosity
of no clinical significance. There are
multiple, small, punctuate areas of
increased density (A) in both hands
and wrists.

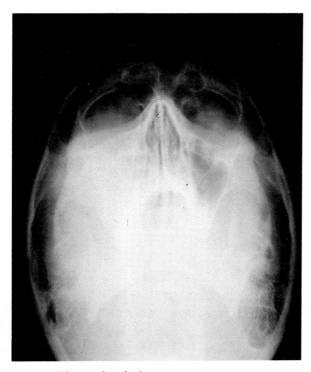

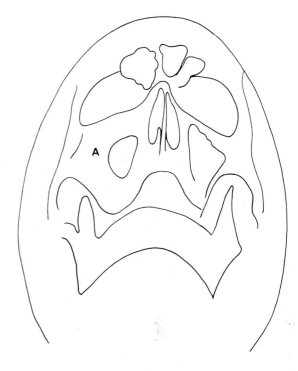

221   Fibrous dysplasia.
In this condition, there is displacement of medullary bone by fibrous tissue. Single (monostotic) or multiple (polyostotic) cyst-like lesions with well-defined walls are formed within bone. They may cause thinning, expansion and pathological fracture. Fibrous dysplasia may occur at any age but is commonest in the first two decades.

(a)   Skull—occipito-mental view.
As well as fibrous lesions, bone forming lesions may occur, particularly in the skull. In this example, marked thickening of the walls of the right maxillary antrum (A) is seen on the occipito-mental view. This type of fibrous dysplasia is sometimes called leontiasis ossea.

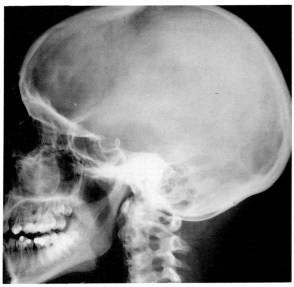

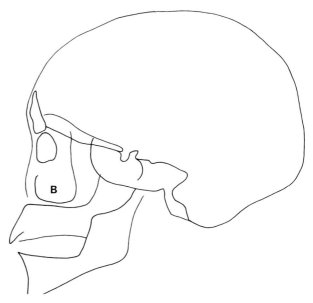

(b)   Lateral view of skull.
A lateral skull view of the same patient shows the thickened maxilla (B) in a different projection.

259

222   Fibrous dysplasia.

(a)   Tibia.
There is an expansile,
relatively radiolucent
lesion (A) with
well-defined margins
(B) arising in the tibial
shaft and expanding it,
thinning the cortex (C).

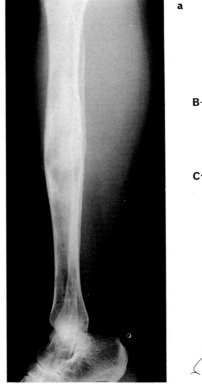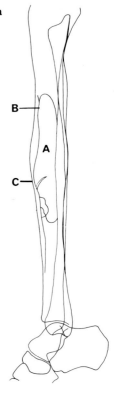

*(b)   Fibrous dysplasia of the
femur in the same patient.*
There is deformity of the
proximal third of the
femur with radiolucent
(A) and sclerotic areas
(B). These are due to
healing of fractures.
Such deformity is
known as the
'shepherd's crook' or
'gnarled stick'
deformity.

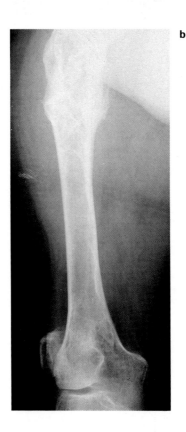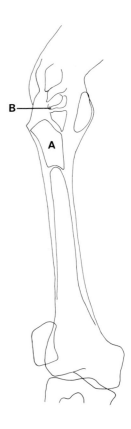

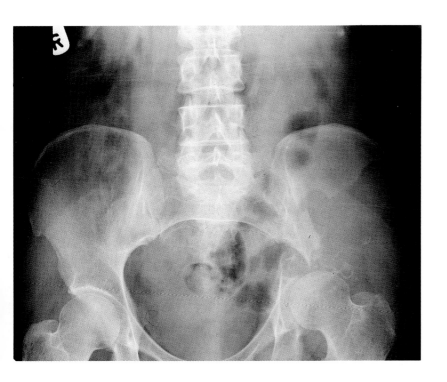

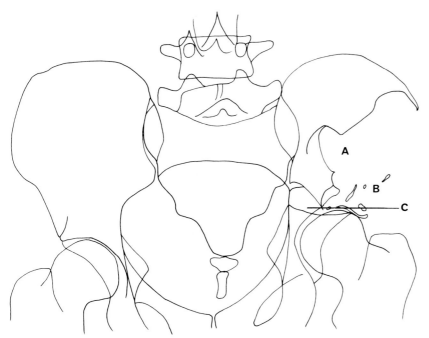

223 **Fibrous dysplasia of pelvis.**
There is a large, expansile lesion (A) with poorly defined borders (B) and a pathological fracture (C).
Fibrous dysplasia may mimic a benign bone cyst or tumour, but in this case it is difficult to distinguish it from a large, destructive metastatic tumour.

224   Neurofibromatosis.
This is a congenital disorder of mesodermal and neuroectodermal tissues. It is recognised clinically by the presence of cutaneous neurofibromata, 'café-au-lait' patches of skin pigmentation and skeletal deformities. These are too varied and widespread to allow full description in an atlas and the reader is referred to larger texts. However, spinal anomalies, particularly kyphosis, occur and soft tissue neurofibromata may cause erosion of bone.

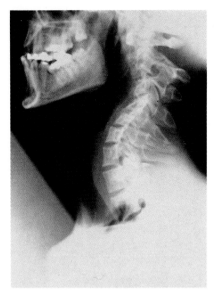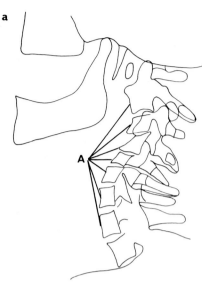

(a)   *Lateral view—cervical spine.*
This example shows cervical spinal kyphosis with abnormal vertebrae (A).

(b)   *AP view—thoracic spine.*
In the thoracic spine of the same patient there is only a mild scoliosis (B).

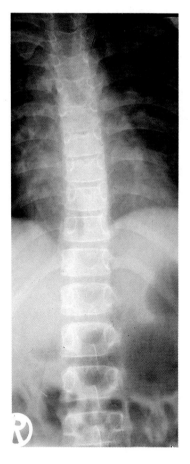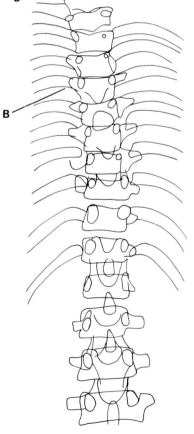

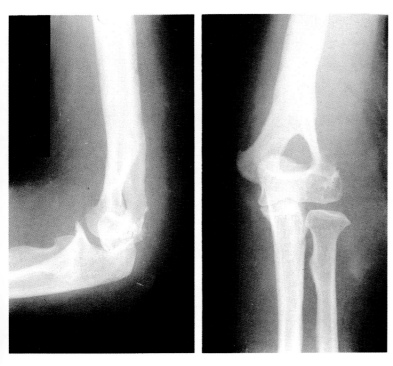

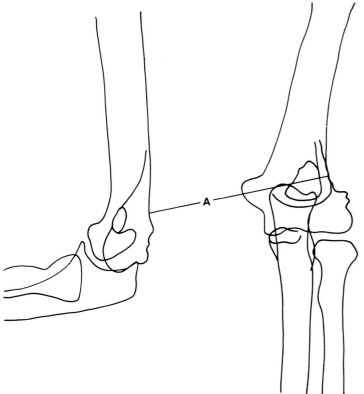

225   Neurofibromatosis of the left elbow.
There is bony erosion of the distal humerus (A) by extrinsic neurofibromata.

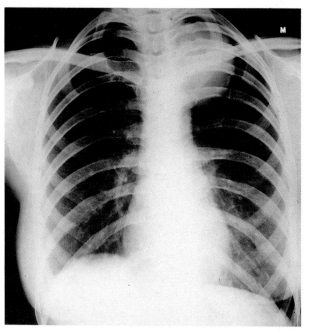
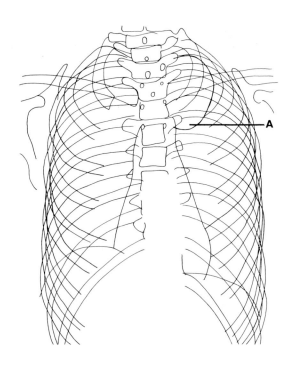

226   Neurofibroma.
There is a solitary thoracic paraspinal neurofibroma presenting as a left posterior mediastinal mass (A).

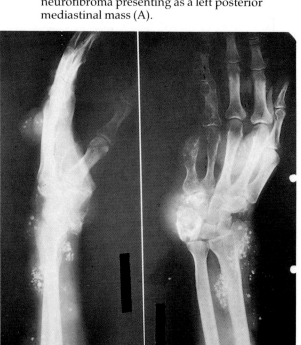
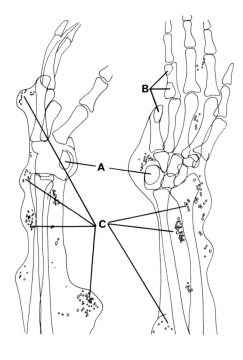

227   Maffucci's syndrome.
Multiple enchondromatosis and cavernous haemangioma. The enchondromata are indistinguishable from those of Ollier's disease (see Bone Tumour section). This film of the forearm, wrist and hand shows expanded enchondromata in the carpus (A) and fourth and fifth digits (B). There are calcified phleboliths (C) in the large cavernous haemangioma, giving rise to extensive soft tissue swelling of the forearm, wrist and hand.

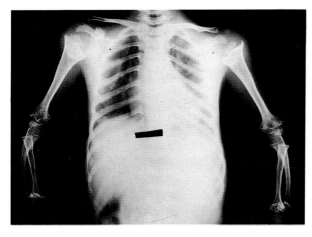

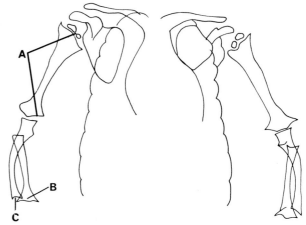

228   Metaphyseal dyschondroplasia (formerly metaphyseal dysostosis).
This comprises a group of rare familial disorders of metaphyseal ossification. The main features are of widened, cupped metaphyses and shortened long bones. There is a resemblance to rickets, particularly in the milder forms, but serum biochemistry is normal.

(a)   AP view—shoulders and arms.
This example shows cupped humeral (A), radial (B) and ulnar metaphyses (C).

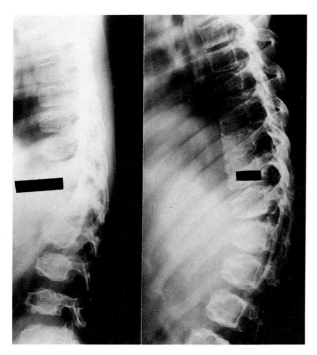

(b)   Lateral views—spine.
The same patient, showing changes in the spinal apophyses (A). At this stage, the combined appearance of metaphyseal changes in the long bones and spinal changes could be designated spondylo-metaphyseal dysplasia.

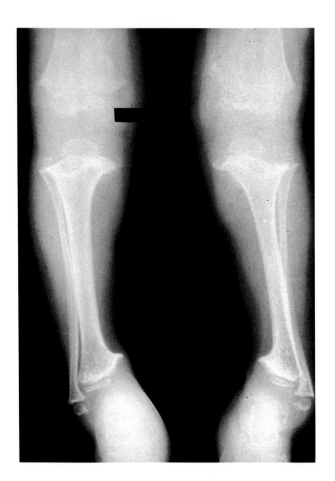 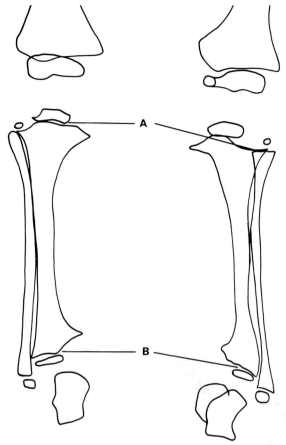

(c) *AP view—legs.*
The same patient, showing metaphyseal
chondrodysplasia of the lower legs.
Metaphyseal flaring is most marked in the
upper (A) and lower tibiae (B).

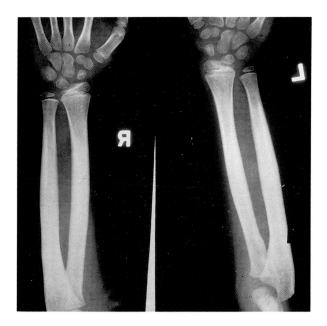

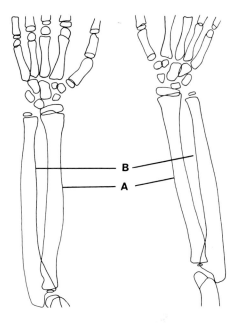

229   Progressive diaphyseal dysplasia (Engelmann's disease).
This condition is limited to the diaphyses of bones, mainly long bones. It is characterised by progressive periosteal and endosteal new bone formation, widening the bone and eventually obliterating the medullary cavities.

(a)   Forearms.
In this example, widening of the diaphyses of the radius (A) and ulna (B) is seen.

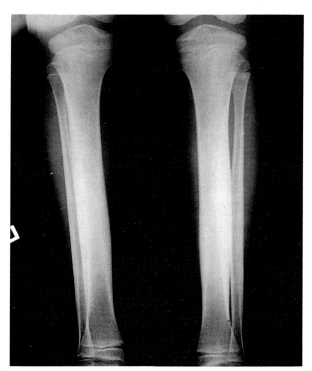

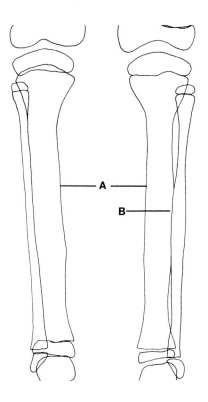

(b)   Lower legs.
Widening of diaphyses of tibiae (A) and fibula (B) in the same patient.

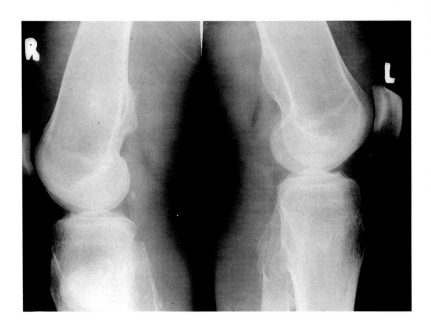

230 Diaphyseal aclasia.
This condition is characterised by the presence of multiple osteochondromata (cartilage-capped exostoses) arising from the ends of the diaphyses close to the metaphyses. The osteochondromata may be polypoid or relatively flat (sessile). The ends of polypoid exostoses always point away from the adjacent joint. Malignant change may occur in less than 10 per cent of cases.

(a) Diaphyseal aclasia of the knee.
The exostoses arise from the distal femora (A) and proximal tibiae (B) and fibulae (C). They point away from the knee. A calcified cap (D) can be seen. The cartilage cap can only be seen if it calcifies.

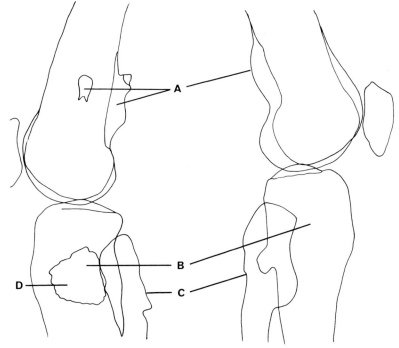

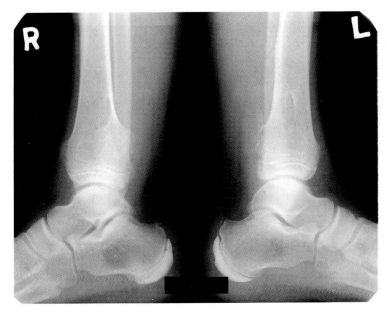

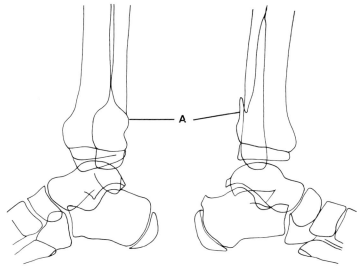

(b) *Both ankles of the same
     patient.*
     Exostoses of the distal
     tibiae are shown (A).

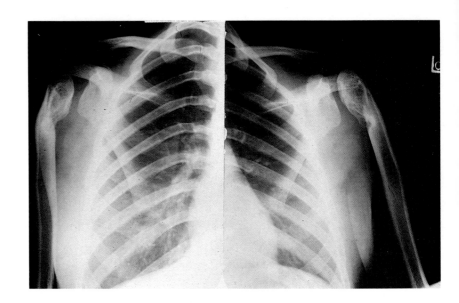

231   Dysplasia epiphysialis multiplex.
In affected sites, commonly hips, knees, ankles, shoulders, elbows and wrists, epiphyses appear late and are small, irregular and fragmented. Any metaphyseal changes are secondary. Premature degenerative joint change may supervene.

(a) *AP view—shoulders.* This example shows flattened proximal humeral epiphyses (A) with secondary deformity of the metaphyses (B). This radiograph has been taken after epiphyseal fusion.

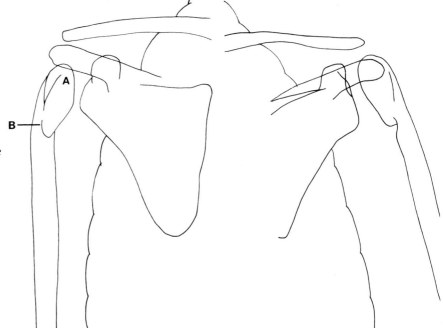

270

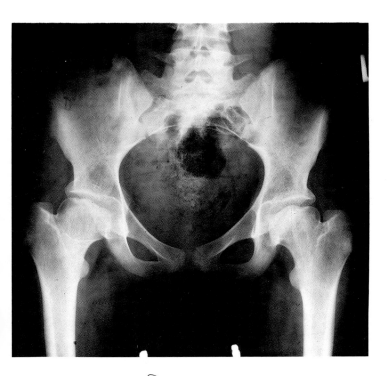

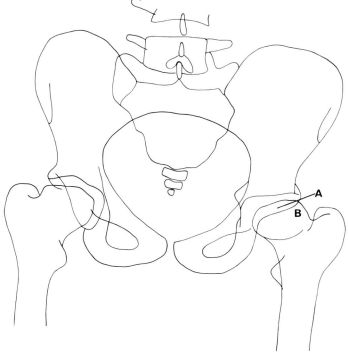

(b) *Pelvis and hips of the same patient.*
There is deformity of the proximal femoral epiphyses (A) and secondary metaphyseal widening (B).

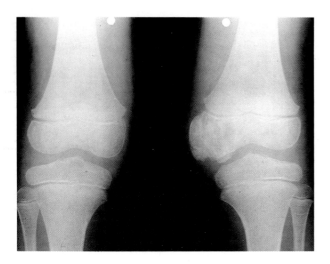

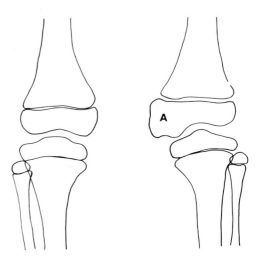

232   Dysplasia epiphysialis hemimelica.
There is overgrowth of one side of an epiphysis (usually medial) with deformity of the adjacent joint. Usually only one joint is affected and the lower limb is predominantly involved. This example shows expansion of the medial side of the distal femoral epiphysis (A).

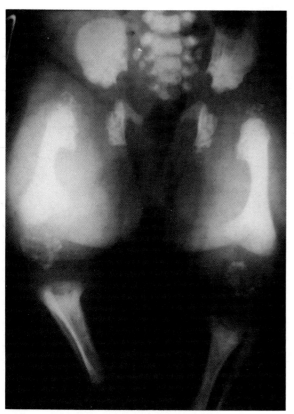

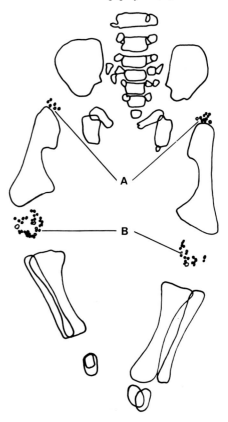

233   Dysplasia epiphysialis punctata (chondrodysplasia punctata).
The epiphyses show multiple punctate increases in density, giving a stippled appearance to the proximal (A) and distal femoral epiphyses (B). Multiple joints are affected and the spine tends to be involved as well as the limb joints.

Other congenital abnormalities may be associated, including mental retardation.

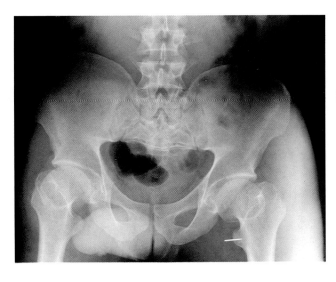

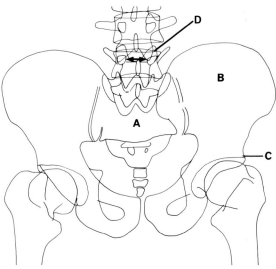

234 **Achondroplasia.**
The achondroplastic is the classic circus
dwarf. The dwarf is short limbed. The
proximal limb bones (humerus and femur)
are more affected than the distal ones. The
skull has a short base.

(a) *AP view—pelvis.*
In the pelvis, the sacrum (A) is narrow, the
ilia (B) are square-shaped and the
acetabular roofs (C) are horizontal. The
spinal interpedicular distance reduces
distally and, in this example, a narrow L5
interpedicular distance can be seen (D).

(b) *Humerus.*
The humeral shaft (A) is
shortened. It appears
relatively wide only
because it is reduced in
length.

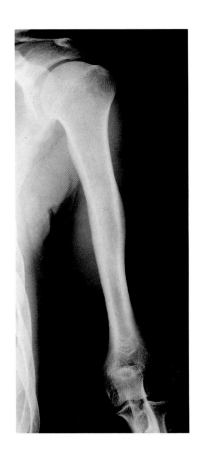

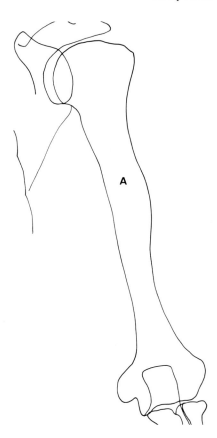

273

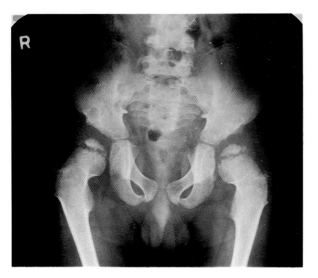

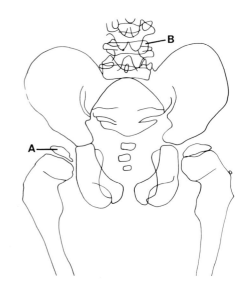

235 **Morquio Brailsford dystrophy (mucopolysaccharidosis IV).**
Biochemically, this condition is included in the mucopolysaccharidoses. Clinically and radiologically, the disorder may remain unnoticed until the child begins weight bearing. The spine shows flattening of the vertebral bodies with thoraco-lumbar kyphosis. A central 'tongue' of bone may be seen protruding forwards from a vertebra. This is secondary to hypoplasia of the antero-superior and inferior corners.

Epiphyseal and metaphyseal deformities occur in long bones. The pelvis in malformed with flaring of the ilia.

(a) *AP view—pelvis.*
This example shows a small, dysplastic proximal femoral epiphysis (A) with flattening (platyspondyly) of the lower lumbar vertebrae (B).

(b) *The same patient—lateral thoraco-lumbar spine showing kyphosis.*
Both the upper and lower vertebral surface are defective and a 'tongue' of bone (A) protrudes anteriorly.

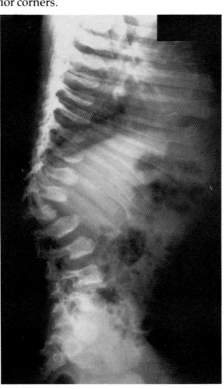

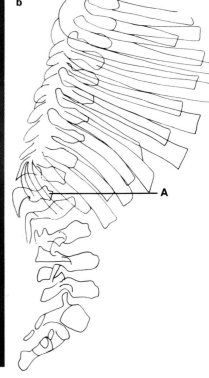

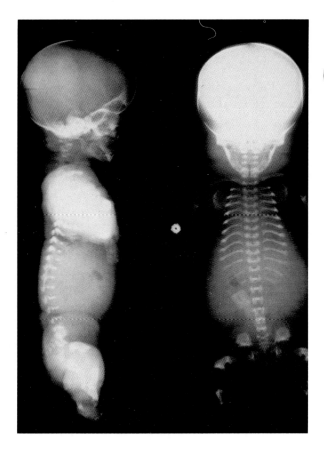
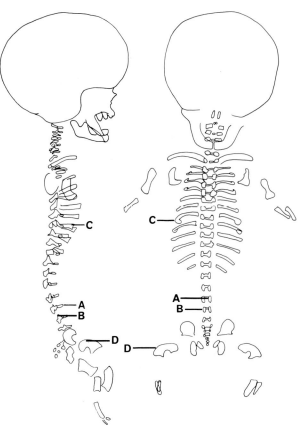

236   **Thanatophoric dwarf.**

As the name suggests, this dwarf is either still-born or dies from asphyxia within the first few hours or days of life. Recognition *in utero* from an ante-natal radiograph is often possible.

This example shows many of the characteristic features. The vertebral bodies (A) are flattened with normal posterior arches (B) rendering the vertebrae H-shaped. The thorax is narrow with short ribs (C). The tubular bones are short and bowed, the shape of the femur resembling a telephone receiver (D).

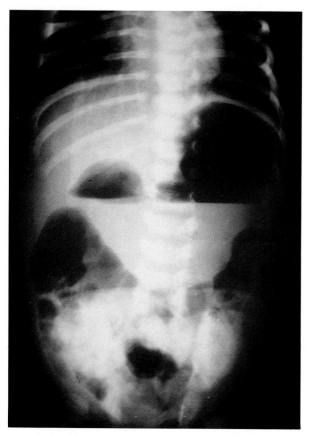

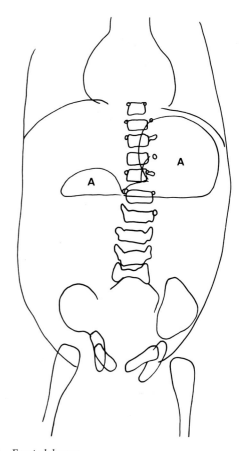

237   Down's syndrome (mongolism).
The clinical features of this condition are characteristic and radiology is not necessary to make the diagnosis. However, radiological abnormalities may be found.

(a)   Erect abdomen.
This film shows a 'double bubble appearance' (A). The larger bubble represents the stomach and the smaller, the dilated proximal duodenum. The appearances are due to duodenal atresia which occurs in Down's syndrome.

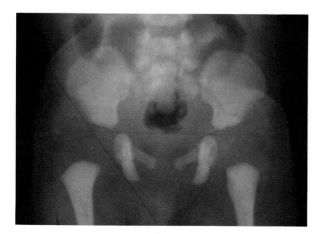

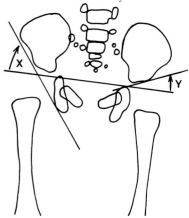

(b)   AP view—pelvis.
A closer look at the pelvis of the same patient shows flattening of the iliac (X) and acetabular angles (Y). The addition of these angles gives the iliac index. If it is under 60 degrees, mongolism is likely. If it is over 78 degrees, mongolism is unlikely.

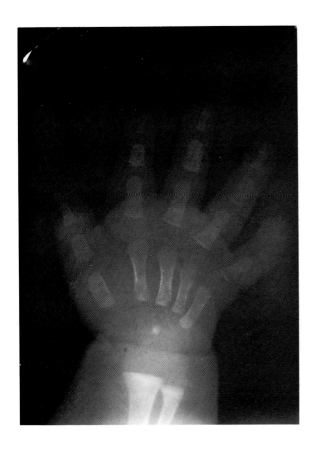

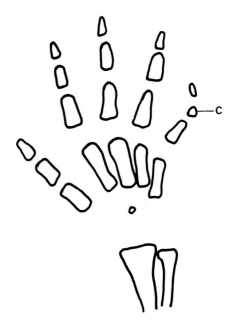

(c) *Hand.*

The hands shows clinodactyly. There is a short, wedged 5th middle phalanx (C). This may also occur as an isolated congenital anomaly in normal individuals.

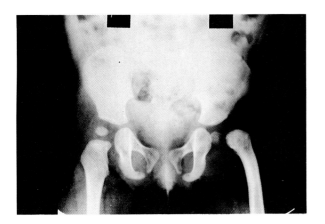

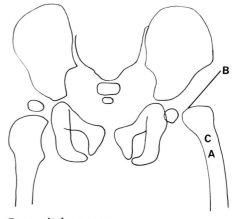

238 **Congenital coxa vara.**

This usually appears soon after birth and is associated with a short, bowed femur (A). The angle between the femoral neck (B) and shaft (C) is more acute than 120 degrees.

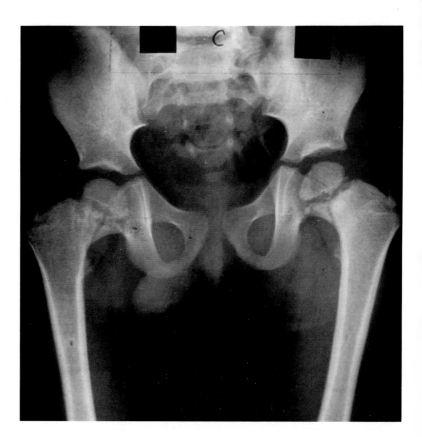

239   Infantile coxa vara.
This usually develops after
birth. It is not truly
congenital and may have a
traumatic aetiology. There
is usually bilateral varus
deformity. This case shows
well-developed bilateral
deformity (A). Triangular
fragments of bone are seen
on the infero-medial
aspects of the femoral necks
(B). This is a characteristic
feature and may be due to
stress fracture.

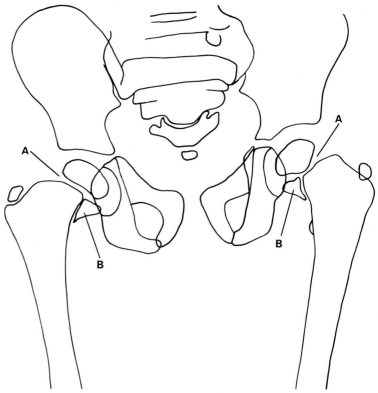

Further Reading

The following books have been helpful to the authors in compiling the text and are recommended to the reader who wishes to consider any of the subjects in greater depth.

CAFFEY J 1978 *Pediatric X-Ray Diagnosis* 7th Edition Year Book Medical Publishers
MURRAY R O and JACKSON H G 1977 *The Radiology of Skeletal Disorders* 2nd Edition Churchill Livingstone
NEVIASER R J, EISENFIELD L S, WIESEL S W and LEWIS R J 1985 *Emergency Orthopaedic Radiology* Churchill Livingstone
SUTTON D 1987 *A Textbook of Radiology and Imaging* 4th Edition Churchill Livingstone
WEIR J and ABRAHAMS P 1986 *An Atlas of Radiological Anatomy* 2nd Edition Churchill Livingstone

INDEX